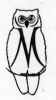

Mastering
Business Letter Writing

Solomon Wiener

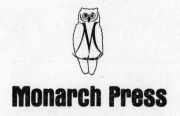

Monarch Press

Published by
Monarch Press
A Simon & Schuster Division of
Gulf & Western Corporation
Simon & Schuster Building
1230 Avenue of the Americas
New York, N.Y. 10020

This is a revised and updated edition of
Business Letter Writing.

Manufactured in the United States of America

10 9 8 7 6 5 4 3 2 1

ISBN: 0-671-18094-0

Dedication

To my family — Gertrude, Marjorie Diane and Willa Kay — in appreciation of their encouragement, understanding and assistance in the numerous tasks required in the preparation of this work.

Preface

In one way or another, all of us belong to the business community. Modern business correspondence consists essentially of business letters—the principal means of commercial communication. It is important for all of us to become proficient in writing business letters.

This book is intended as a concise, practical guide for writing correct and effective business letters, and as a handy manual for quick and convenient reference. You will find it easy to become proficient in writing business letters by first learning and then applying the fundamental principles and techniques presented in this book.

Following this Preface is a detailed table of contents. Note that all facets of modern business correspondence—the mechanics, the different styles and kinds of letters, good grammar and correct usage in letter writing, and even the social-personal aspects of business communications are discussed clearly and concisely.

A great deal of related information is also given. There are sections on Mailgram messages, telegrams and other telegraphic services; greeting cards as good-will instruments; special forms of address for officials; commonly used abbreviations, signs and symbols; and other pertinent matter. Throughout the book, there are many sample letters, illustrations and sample telegram messages to support the text material, numerous reviews for reinforcing knowledge as it is acquired, and practice exercises for self-testing and further review.

Read this book. Study it. Keep it handy, at the office, at home, in school. Refer to it as often as necessary. Do become proficient in the art of writing correct and effective business letters.

Solomon Wiener

New York, New York

Contents

GENERAL INFORMATION REGARDING
   BUSINESS LETTERS 1
Stationery 1
The Letterhead 2
The Continuing Sheet 2
The Message-Reply Form 2
The Aerogramme 2
Spacing and Punctuation 3
The Different Styles of Business Letters 3
   Full Block Style 3
   Block Style 4
   Semi-block Style 4
   Simplified Style 4
   Hanging Indentation Style.. 4
   Indented Style 5

THE ESSENTIAL PARTS OF THE BUSINESS LETTER 6
The Heading 6
The Inside Address 6
The Salutation 7
The Body of the Letter 7
The Complimentary Closing 7
The Signature 7

SOME SPECIAL FEATURES OF THE
   BUSINESS LETTER 10
The Personal Notation.. 10
The Reference Line 10
The Attention Line 10
The Subject Line 10
The Identification Line 10
The Enclosure Notation 11
The Mailing Notation 11
The Carbon Copy Distribution Notation 11
The Postscript 11

ADDRESSING THE ENVELOPE 13

FOLDING AND INSERTING THE LETTER............................ 15

THE DIFFERENT KINDS OF BUSINESS LETTERS 17
Letters of General Inquiry 17
   The Letter Requesting a Favor 17

The Letter Answering a Request for a Favor 17
The Letter of Inquiry Regarding a Possible Purchase 20
Suggested Answers to a Possible Buyer 20
Sales Letters 23
Letters Regarding Credit and Credit Standing 27
Letter from an Individual Requesting Credit 27
Letter Acknowledging Credit Request from an Individual 28
Letter Granting Credit to an Individual 28
Letter Refusing Credit to an Individual 28
Letter from a Firm That Has Just Bought a Business and
    Asks for a Continuance of Credit Previously Given 29
Letters Regarding Orders to Be Sent on Open Account 29
Letters Regarding Credit Standing 31
Letters Regarding Orders 34
Letters Regarding Remittances 39
Letters Regarding Past Due Accounts 42
Letters of Complaint and Adjustment 44
Letters Regarding Employment 48
Applying for the Position 48
Acknowledging the Letter of Application 48
Follow-up by the Applicant 50
Checking References... 50

MISCELLANEOUS LETTERS ON THE SOCIAL-
PERSONAL ASPECTS OF MODERN BUSINESS 53
Accepting or Declining an Invitation to Deliver an Address.. 53
Acknowledging a Letter That Is Being Referred to
    Someone Else for Reply 53
Cancelling an Appointment 53
Changing the Address for a Subscription 55
Confirming a Hotel Reservation 55
Congratulating a Friend on his Promotion............................. 55
Explaining a Delay in Answering a Letter 55
Extending Holiday Greetings... 56
Introducing a Person by Letter 58
Making a Hotel Reservation 58
Ordering Theater Tickets 60
Submitting a Letter of Resignation 60

MAILGRAMS, TELEGRAMS, AND OTHER
TELEGRAPHIC SERVICES 61
Domestic Telegraph Service... 61
Mailgram Messages 61
Telegrams.. 61
Format for Domestic Telegraph Blanks 63
Preparing the Telegraph Form for Transmission 63
Telegraphic Money Orders 63
Teletypewriters... 66
Facsimile 66
Business Correspondence by Telegraph 67
Special Social and Other Domestic Telegraph Services 67
International Telegraph Service 69
Format for International Telegraph Blanks............................. 69
Preparing the Telegraph Form for Transmission 69

GOOD GRAMMAR AND CORRECT USAGE
IN LETTER WRITING 72
The Parts of Speech 72
   Nouns 72
   Pronouns 72
   Adjectives 74
   Verbs 74
      Agreement of the Verb with the Subject................ 74
      The Different Moods of the Verb....................... 75
      Use and Formation of Tenses 75
      Principal Parts of Irregular and Other Special Verbs.......... 77
   Adverbs 80
   Prepositions 80
   Conjunctions 80
   Interjections.. 80
Phrases, Clauses and Sentences 80
   The Phrase 80
   The Clause 80
   The Sentence 81
      Parts of the Sentence 81
Rules of Spelling 81
Other Troublesome Words.. 83
Trite or Hackneyed Words and Expressions................. 87
Rules for Dividing Words... 87
Rules of Punctuation... 88
Rules of Capitalization 91
The Use of Contractions 92

MISCELLANEOUS INFORMATION 93
Special Forms of Address for Officials 93
   Public Officials 93
   School Officials and Faculty 96
   Members of the Clergy 98
   Members of the Armed Forces 100
Abbreviations of the States, the District of Columbia
and Possessions of the United States 105
Other Commonly Used Abbreviations......................... 106
Commonly Used Signs and Symbols........................... 109

General Information Regarding Business Letters

Stationery

The paper and envelopes used in business correspondence are known as *stationery*. The most commonly used size of letterhead paper is 8½ by 11 inches. The half sheet used for very short letters is 5½ by 8½ inches. Stationery used for air mail to foreign countries is generally light in weight to save postage.

For the more personal type of business letter, many executives and professional offices use the *Monarch* or *Executive* size, a sheet 7¼ by 10½ inches.

The envelopes used with these different sizes of letter papers are:

The *No. 10 envelope* fits the standard size letter of 8½ by 11 inches. This type of envelope is 4⅛ by 9½ inches. It is commonly known as the large commercial envelope.

The *No. 6¾ envelope* measures 3⅝ by 6½ inches. It is used with half sheets, standard letter-size sheets and some personal-type business letters. It is commonly known as the small commercial envelope.

The *No. 7 envelope* for the *Monarch* or *Executive* size letter sheet measures 3⅞ by 7½ inches.

Other sizes of business envelopes are:

No. 12	4¾ by 11 inches
No. 11	4½ by 10⅜ inches
No. 9	3⅞ by 8⅞ inches
No. 8⅝	3⅝ by 8⅝ inches
No. 7¾	3⅞ by 7½ inches
No. 6¼	3½ by 6 inches

Business reply and return address envelopes come in many different sizes; however, the No. 6¾, No. 7 and No. 9 are the most widely used.

The *window envelope* has a transparent inset through which the address can be seen; the open panel envelope has an opening without such inset. These envelopes are rarely used for formal business letters but are generally used for mailing invoices, purchase orders, checks, notices, receipts, etc. They are also used with the informal message-reply forms. The double-window envelopes are used to show the addresses of both the receiver and the sender.

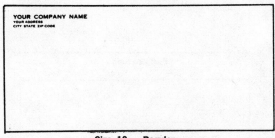

Size 10 — Regular

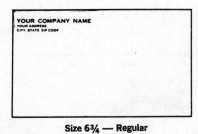

Size 6¾ — Regular

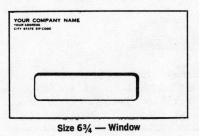

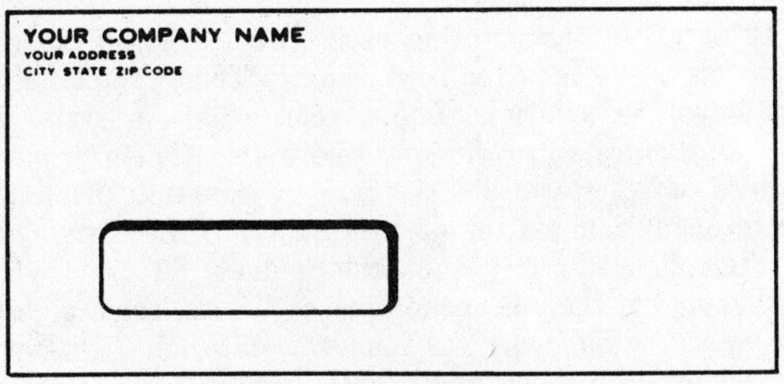

Size 10 — Window

Size 6¾ — Window

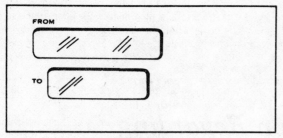

Double window

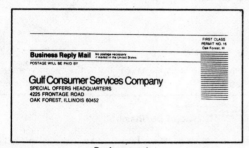

FIRST CLASS
PERMIT NO. 15
Oak Forest, Ill.

Business Reply Mail No postage necessary if mailed in the United States
POSTAGE WILL BE PAID BY

Gulf Consumer Services Company
SPECIAL OFFERS HEADQUARTERS
4225 FRONTAGE ROAD
OAK FOREST, ILLINOIS 60452

Business reply

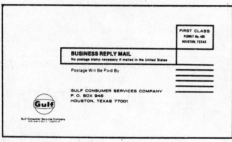

FIRST CLASS
PERMIT No. 485
HOUSTON, TEXAS

BUSINESS REPLY MAIL
No postage stamp necessary if mailed in the United States

Postage Will Be Paid By

Gulf

GULF CONSUMER SERVICES COMPANY
P. O. BOX 946
HOUSTON, TEXAS 77001

Return envelope

The letterhead

The style of the printing used on a letterhead depends largely on the taste of the firm using it. Today, the tendency is to have the printing simple, yet modern in style. The name and address are the only really essential information required on a letterhead. All other information printed on a letterhead is a matter of preference. Some firms have their telephone number and cable address on their letterhead; some list their branches and affiliates; some give the year when the business was founded; and some firms print separate letterheads for their officers, executives or departments. However, when a business has its own corporate symbol or slogan, it always appears on the letterhead.

The continuing sheet

Most business letters rarely exceed one page. If a letter requires more than one page, use a "continuing sheet" of the same color, weight and quality as the letterhead. A letterhead must never be used for the continuing sheet. Each page of a letter beyond the first page should be numbered consecutively. The name of the addressee, the page number

and the date of the letter should appear at the top of each continuing sheet.

The message-reply form

To cut down correspondence costs, many concerns are using the three-part, carbon-interleaved message-reply form for internal correspondence and for short, informal business notes. The messages may be handwritten or typewritten and are used for sending short memos, making inquiries, following up orders, writing to salesmen, etc.

The form is generally 8½ by 7 inches (without the stub). The top sheet is white; the second copy is yellow; the third copy is pink. After the message is written or typed, the sender removes the yellow copy for filing and possible follow up, and sends out the top sheet with carbon and triplicate (pink) copy in a window envelope. The recipient writes or types a reply in the reply section of the form, separates the copies and sends the top sheet with the original message and reply back. This procedure enables both parties to have identical records of the original message and the reply.

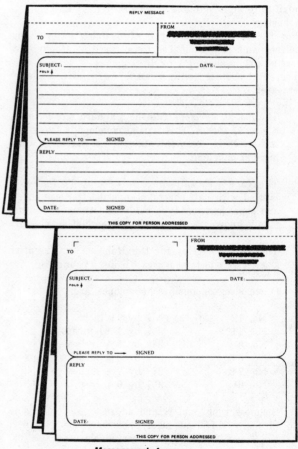

Message-reply forms

The aerogramme

Available at all post offices, the aerogramme provides the most economical means of sending a letter by airmail to all parts of the world. Approximately 7¼ by 10½ inches of message area are available on the blank side and 7¼ by 3½ inches of additional message area are available on the lower third of the printed side. After the message is written, the aerogramme sheet is folded into the form of an envelope and is then sealed.

Although aerogrammes are used principally for personal messages, they may also be used for informal business notes. However, no enclosures are permitted.

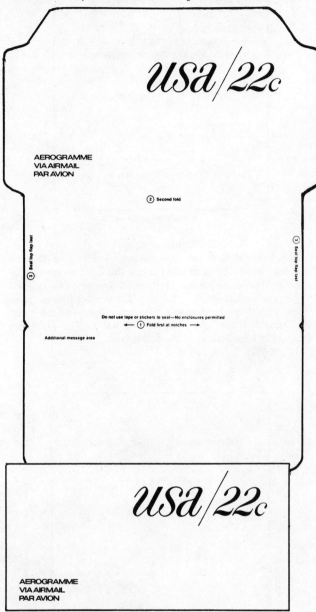

Spacing and punctuation

The inside address of a letter is usually typed single space. The body of the letter should also be single spaced, with double spacing between the paragraphs. If, however, the letter is very short and the paragraphs are indented, the body of the letter may be double spaced to improve the appearance of the letter.

A letter may be punctuated in *closed*, *open* or *mixed* style. *Closed punctuation* requires punctuation marks after the date line, each line of the inside address, the complimentary closing and each line of the signature. *Open punctuation* does not require any punctuation marks unless it is necessary to ab-

breviate a word at the end of a line. *Mixed punctuation*, the preferred style today, is a modification of open punctuation. It requires a colon after the salutation and a comma after the complimentary closing.

Closed Punctuation	*Open Punctuation*	*Mixed Punctuation*
March 5, 19......	March 5, 19......	March 5, 19......
Mr. Thomas Scott, 350 Elm Street, Dayton, Ohio 45401	Mr. Thomas Scott 350 Elm Street Dayton, Ohio 45401	Mr. Thomas Scott 350 Elm Street Dayton, Ohio 45401
Dear Mr. Scott:	Dear Mr. Scott	Dear Mr. Scott:
Sincerely yours,	Sincerely yours	Sincerely yours,
John Forman	*John Forman*	*John Forman*
John Forman, Credit Manager	John Forman Credit Manager	John Forman Credit Manager

The different styles of business letters

Business letters may be arranged in several different styles. It is customary for a business concern to adopt one style for its letters, thereby making it easier to associate the particular style with the firm. The following forms of letter arrangements are in current use:

Full block style   Simplified style
Block style   Hanging indentation style
Semi-block style   Indented style

Examples of the different styles of business letters follow.

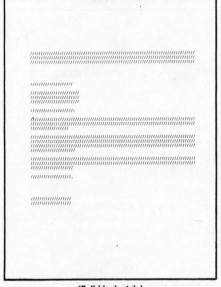

(Full block style)

Full block style

In the full block style, all parts of the letter start flush with the left-hand margin. There are no indentations. Open punctuation is frequently used. This style is gaining in popularity.

3

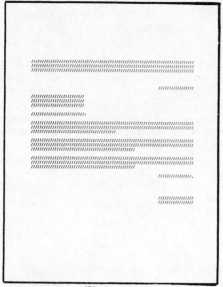

(Block style)

Block style

The block style has been in use for a long time. In this style, the inside address and the paragraphs are blocked flush with the left-hand margin, as is the salutation. The dateline is flush with the right-hand margin. The blocked signature is aligned with the complimentary closing. This style is one of the most popular letter styles today.

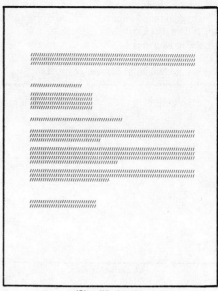

(Simplified style)

Simplified style

This letter style is based on the full block style with open punctuation. In this simplified style, the salutation and the complimentary closing are omitted. A subject line is used but the word *SUBJECT* is deleted. The subject line is typed in capital letters three spaces below the inside address and three spaces above the body of the letter. The signature line is typed four spaces below the body.

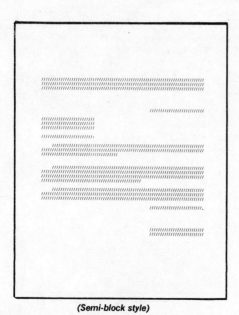

(Semi-block style)

Semi-block style

This popular but somewhat conservative style is similar to the indented style except for the blocked inside address and the blocked signature portion which is aligned with the complimentary closing.

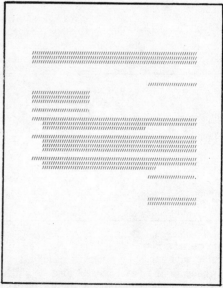

(Hanging indentation style)

Hanging indentation style

The hanging indentation style is not generally used in routine business correspondence. It is used in advertising letters to attract particular attention. In this style, the first line of each paragraph is flush with the left-hand margin. The other lines are generally indented five spaces.

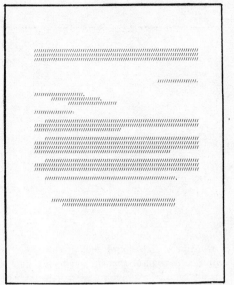

(Indented style)

Indented style

In this conservative style, each line of the inside address is indented five spaces more than the preceding line. The first line of each paragraph in the body of the letter is generally indented five spaces. The signature is not aligned with the complimentary closing but is indented five spaces. Closed punctuation is generally used in the inside address, as well as after the date line and signature. This style is rarely used today.

REVIEW

1. When do we use a light weight paper and envelope?
2. What are the dimensions of the standard letter sheet?
3. What are the dimensions of the half sheet?
4. What information must appear on a letterhead?
5. Should a letterhead be used for a continuing sheet? Explain.
6. What information should appear at the top of a continuing sheet?
7. What numbers are used to identify (a) the large commercial envelope? (b) the small commercial envelope?
8. What type letter sheet is used with the No. 7 envelope?
9. What size envelope is used in most business correspondence?
10. (a) What do we call an envelope that has a transparent inset? (b) For what purpose do we generally use this type of envelope?
11. What is the usual spacing in a typewritten business letter?
12. How do we space a very short business letter?
13. Explain the difference between *open* and *closed* punctuation.
14. What is the preferred type of punctuation in a business letter?
15. What are the characteristics of the indented style of letter?
16. Name the styles of letter arrangement in which all parts start flush with the left-hand margin.
17. What are the characteristics of the popular block style?
18. How does the semi-block style differ from the block style?
19. What are the characteristics of the simplified style?
20. For what purpose is the hanging indentation style of letter used?

The Essential Parts of the
Business Letter

Business letters are made up of the following parts:

The heading*	The salutation
(The letterhead	The body of the letter
and date)	The complimentary closing
The inside address	The signature

The different parts of a business letter are arranged in the following manner:

////////////////////// LETTERHEAD* //////////////////////

////////////// DATE //////////////

//// INSIDE ADDRESS ////

// SALUTATION //:

////////////// BODY //////////////

// COMPLIMENTARY CLOSING //,
SIGNATURE

The heading (the letterhead and date)
The heading on the stationery of most business firms is printed, showing the name and address. The date is typed in at least two spaces below the last line of the letterhead. The exact position of the date depends on the design of the letterhead and the style in which the letter is typed.

It is seldom that a business firm does not have a printed letterhead. However, when a printed letterhead is not available, the heading (complete address and date) must be

*In the absence of a letterhead, the heading consists of the address and date.

typed in the upper right-hand part of the letter sheet, with at least an inch margin at the top and to the right as shown:

```
                    2108 Washington Avenue
                    Louisville, KY  40103
                    September 27,  19__
```

Where an address has to be typed in, the words *avenue, street,* etc., are not abbreviated. Numbered streets up to ten are spelled out, while numbered streets beyond ten are written in figures. Do not use *st, nd* or *d, rd,* or *th* when figures are used for numbered streets or for the days of the month in dates. The names of cities or towns must be written in full. The names of states or possessions should be abbreviated if there is a lack of space; the District of Columbia is generally abbreviated. Be sure to include the ZIP Code on all addresses. Special 2-letter abbreviations authorized by the U.S. Postal Service for the names of states, the District of Columbia and United States possessions are listed on page 190. Do not abbreviate the name of the month in the date line and be certain to place a comma between the day of the month and the year.

The inside address
The inside address gives the name and address of the firm or individual to whom the letter is addressed. It is placed at the left-hand side of the sheet, at least two spaces below the heading. The inside address must occupy at least three lines. If the individual or firm has no street address, type the city and state on separate lines. The exact position of the inside address depends on the length of the letter and the size of the sheet. The following is an example showing where the inside address appears in relation to the printed letterhead.

```
//////////////////////////////////
/////////// LETTERHEAD ///////////
//////////////////////////////////


                        //// DATE ////

Current Fashions, Inc.
5 West 38 Street
New York, N.Y. 10018
```

Regardless of the style used in typing a business letter, such words as *Mr., Mrs., Miss, Ms., Dr., Dean, General*, etc., must always appear *before* the name. Where the person addressed has an official or business title, this should appear *after* the name, either next to it or on the following line. Do not abbreviate official or business titles. If there is an apartment, room, or suite number, it should be placed immediately after the street address on the same line.

Here are examples of the proper forms of inside address to individuals:

Mr. William Morgan, Treasurer
Regents Furniture Company
210 Park Avenue South
New York, New York   10003

Mr. George Finster
Director of Public Relations
American Paint Manufacturing Co.
645 Fifth Avenue
New York, New York   10019

Dr. Edward Russell
Industrial Chemical Corp.
312 Central Avenue
New Brunswick, NJ   08901

Employment Manager
Nassau Pharmaceutical Co., Room 401
5042 Grand Avenue
Los Angeles, Calif.   90052

The salutation (or greeting)

This is placed two spaces below the inside address, flush with the left-hand margin. The first and last words and every noun in the salutation are capitalized. A colon follows the salutation in business letters unless open punctuation is used. The example below shows how the salutation looks, following the inside address:

```
/////////////////////
// INSIDE ADDRESS //
/////////////////////

My dear Mr. Smith:
```

Some of the more commonly used forms of salutation are:

Singular (to an individual)	*Masculine*	*Feminine*
	Dear Sir:*	Dear Madam:*
	My dear Mr. Ford:	My dear Mrs. Ford:
	Dear Mr. Ford:	Dear Ms. Ford:
(Entirely Personal)	Dear William:	Dear Gertrude:
	Dear Bill:	Dear Trudy:
Plural (to a company or association)	Gentlemen:	Mesdames:

*This form of salutation is used when the name of the person is not known.

The body of the letter

The body is the most important part of the letter. A business letter should be clear, concise and to the point. Greater effectiveness will be achieved if these suggestions are followed:

Make sure that the subject matter of the letter is presented in well-organized paragraphs.

Use words that are in common, accepted usage. Avoid slang, colloquialisms or trite expressions.

Be careful of the spelling of words. When in doubt, consult the dictionary.

Use capital letters where necessary and punctuate to make your meaning clear.
See to it that the letter is typed neatly.

It is advisable to keep copies of business letters for future reference.

The complimentary closing

The complimentary closing (the farewell) is placed two spaces below the body of the letter. It appears at the right-hand side of the sheet, except in the full-block style in which it appears at the left-hand margin. It is omitted when the simplified style is used. Only the first word of the complimentary closing is capitalized. A comma is placed at the end, except when open punctuation is used. Example:

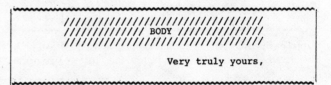

Some of the more commonly used forms of complimentary closings are:

Respectfully,	Sincerely yours,
Respectfully yours,	Yours sincerely,
Yours truly,	Very sincerely,
Yours very truly,	Cordially,
Very truly yours,	Cordially yours,

(Entirely Personal)
Yours,
Your friend,

Some forms of complimentary closings, like the following, are no longer acceptable:

Expecting an early reply, I am,
Hoping to hear from you soon, I remain,
Thanking you in advance, I remain,
I am, obediently yours,
I remain, your humble servant,

The signature

The signature is placed directly below the complimentary closing. It must be handwritten in ink, and legible. No punctuation follows the signature. Titles or degrees, such as *Mr., Rev., M.D., Ph.D.*, etc., are not used with the signature in business letters. However, *Mrs.* or *Miss* may be used.

The name of the person who is signing the letter is typed four spaces below the complimentary closing. If the simplified style is used, the complimentary closing is omitted, and the signature line is typed four spaces below the body. An official title, if used, is placed directly below the typewritten name.

Sincerely yours,

Fred Collins

Fred Collins

Sincerely yours,

Alfred Clark

Alfred Clark
Manager

A married woman* signs her name as indicated below:

Yours very truly,

Elizabeth D. Harris

Elizabeth D. Harris
(Mrs. Fred C. Harris)

If she so wishes, an unmarried woman writes the word *Ms.* before her typewritten name:

Yours very truly,

May D. Klings

Ms. May D. Klings

In business letters, if the pronoun *we* is used instead of *I*, the name of the firm appears before the writer's signature.

The firm's name is typed two spaces below the complimentary closing followed by the writer's name four spaces below the firm's name.

Very truly yours,

THE AMERICAN TEXTILE Co.

Ralph Higgens

Ralph Higgens
Vice-President

When a secretary signs her employer's name to a letter he dictated, she places her initials directly below the handwritten signature.

Very truly yours,

Paul Carroll *A.S.*

Paul Carroll
Manager

When a secretary signs a letter in her own name, she indicates it as follows:

Yours very truly,

Marjorie D'one

Secretary to Mr. Davis

REVIEW

1. Name the essential parts of the business letter.
2. What must be typed to complete the heading on a letterhead?
3. If a plain sheet of paper is used, what information must appear in the heading?
4. Are cardinal or ordinal numbers employed when figures are used for numbered streets or avenues? Explain.
5. Does the ZIP Code number appear between the names of the city or town and the state? Explain.
6. a. May the name of the city or town be abbreviated in the heading or inside address? Explain.
   b. May the name of the state be abbreviated in the heading or inside address? Explain.
7. May the name of the month be abbreviated in the date line?
8. What punctuation, if any, is placed between the day of the month and the year? Is any punctuation placed between the month and the day of the month?
9. What information is generally contained in the inside address?
10. Does the inside address always follow directly after the date line? Explain.
11. If a letter is being sent to an official of a firm, must his official title appear on the same line with his name? Explain.
12. What words in the salutation must be capitalized?
13. What punctuation is placed after the salutation in business letters when other than open punctuation is used?
14. What kinds of expressions do we try to avoid in writing the body of the letter?
15. How do we arrange the body of the letter in presenting our thoughts?
16. What salutation is used when writing to an individual whose position is known but whose name is not known?
17. What salutation is generally used when writing to a corporation or other large organization?
18. Why is it advisable to make and keep copies of business letters?
19. What word or words in the complimentary closing must be capitalized?
20. What punctuation is placed after the complimentary closing in a business letter when other than open punctuation is used?
21. What punctuation, if any, is placed after the signature?
22. How does a woman indicate in her signature that she is unmarried?
23. How does a woman indicate in her signature that she is married?
24. When does the firm's name appear before the writer's signature in a business letter?
25. How does a secretary indicate that she has signed her employer's name to a letter?

---

*A widow generally signs her name in the same way as a married woman.

8

1. Write the heading to be placed on a plain sheet of paper, based on the following information: The letter is being written today; you live in Boise, Idaho; your street address is 317 Central Avenue; the ZIP Code number is 93701.

2. Write the inside address and appropriate salutation for each of the following:
   a. Mr. Norman Parker, Vice-President, Universal Rubber Co., Inc., 1425 Atlantic Avenue, Youngstown, Ohio, ZIP Code number 44503.
   b. Business Editor, York Magazine, Inc., 21 Duke Circle, Alexandria, Virginia, ZIP Code number 22314.
   c. National Machine Company, 1234 Royden Road, North Hollywood, California, ZIP Code number 91604.
   d. Miss Helen B. Hoffman, 83 Smith Hall, Syracuse University, Syracuse, New York, ZIP Code number 13203.
   e. Dr. Marion Buckley, Director of Research, Commercial Chemicals, 83 Funnel Drive, Kansas City, Missouri, ZIP Code number 64108.

3. Assume that you are Publicity Manager for the Pacific Steamship Company and have just written a routine business letter.
   a. Write an appropriate signature for this letter.
   b. If you used the pronoun *we* frequently, what would be a suitable signature for such a letter?

4. a. A business letter is written by Eileen B. Murray, wife of Richard C. Murray. Write the proper signature for this individual indicating her marital status.
   b. A business letter is written by Louise C. Joyce, an unmarried woman. Write the appropriate signature for this person indicating that she is single.

5. Shirley S. Milner is secretary to Edward Grey, Advertising Manager. Write the appropriate signature for each of the following instances.
   a. The secretary signs her employer's signature to a letter he has dictated.
   b. The secretary signs a letter in her own name.

Some Special Features of the
Business Letter

The personal notation

If your letter is of a confidential nature and you want it read by a particular person only, use the word *personal* or *confidential* to indicate this. Such notation should appear four spaces above the inside address in the letter, as well as on the envelope. Example:

```
                         ////DATE////


    PERSONAL


    ////////////////
    /INSIDE ADDRESS/
    ////////////////
```

The reference line

A *reference line* can refer to a bill, an order, a code or a letter. It is typed four spaces below the date line. Examples:

```
                         ////DATE////

    In reply, refer to File No. 4781
    ////////////////
    /INSIDE ADDRESS/
    ////////////////
```

```
                         ////DATE////


    Refer to File No. 4-ML-X
    ////////////////
    /INSIDE ADDRESS/
    ////////////////
```

The attention line

If, in writing a business letter to a firm, you want it directed to the attention of a particular individual, use the *attention line*. This line is placed a double space below the inside address and a double space above the salutation. It may be flush with the left-hand margin, indented five spaces, or centered. Although the letter is directed to an individual, a plural salutation is required because the letter is addressed to the firm. Example:

```
    ////////////////
    /INSIDE ADDRESS/
    ////////////////

    Attention Mr. George Johnson

    Gentlemen:
```

The subject line

The *subject line* indicates the subject matter of the letter and makes it unnecessary to devote the first paragraph to giving this information. This line is generally centered on the same line with the salutation or two spaces below. If the full block style is used, type the subject line flush with the left-hand margin two spaces below the salutation. Place a colon after the word *Subject* and use initial capital letters for all important words. Example:

```
    SALUTATION


              Subject:  Points for Annual Credit
```

If the simplified style is used, the subject line is typed in all capital letters, but "Subject:" is deleted.

```
    ////////////////////
    /// INSIDE ADDRESS //
    ////////////////////

    POINTS FOR ANNUAL CREDIT
```

The identification line

The *identification line* is made up of the initials of the name of the person who dictated the letter and those of the secretary or typist. The initials may be in all capital letters, in all small letters, or in capitalized letters for the dictator and in small letters for the secretary or typist. It is usually typed two spaces below the signature, flush with the left-hand margin. Example:

```
                                          // SIGNATURE //
        SJW:am
```

The enclosure notation

When a letter has an enclosure, the notation to that effect is typed directly below the identification line, flush with the left-hand margin. Either the entire word *Enclosure*, or its abbreviation, *Enc.* or *Encl.* may be used. If a letter has more than one enclosure the number should be stated. Examples:

```
        SJW:am
        Enclosure
```

```
        SJW:am
        2 Encls.
```

The mailing notation

This notation states the method of mailing: whether a letter is to be sent *registered, airmail, special delivery*, etc. It is typed directly below the identification line or enclosure notation. It serves as a record to indicate that the letter was sent by other than regular mail. Examples:

```
        SJW:am
        Registered
```

```
        SJW:am
        2 Encls.
        Special Delivery
```

The carbon copy distribution notation

This notation states that a carbon copy of the letter is being sent to another person. It is typed two spaces below all other notations, flush with the left-hand margin. Either the words *Copy to* or the abbreviation *cc:* (carbon copy) may be used. Examples:

```
        SJW:am
        Enclosure
        Copy to Mr. J. Nelson
```

```
        SJW:am
        Enc.
        cc: Mr. J. Nelson
```

The blind carbon copy notation (bcc:) is used when the addressor does not wish to indicate the distribution of the carbon copies to the addressee. It is placed on all internal copies, but not on the letter sent to the addressee.

The postscript

This word usually written as P.S. is derived from Latin. It means *written after* and is used in the sense of an afterthought. In most business and personal correspondence it appears two spaces below the identification line or the last notation, in the same style as the letter. The abbreviation *P.S.* is the accepted form, but the use of the notation itself is entirely optional. When the notation is used, however, the initials of the person who dictated appear below the postscript. Example:

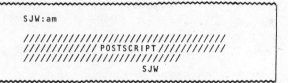

```
        SJW:am

        ///////////////////////////////////
        /////////// POSTSCRIPT /////////////
        ///////////////////////////////
                                          SJW
```

REVIEW

1. What does the personal notation in a letter indicate? Where is this notation typed?
2. Where, in addition to the business letter, does the personal notation appear?
3. What does a reference line refer to? Where is this line typed?
4. What purpose does the attention line serve? Where is it typed? In a letter that has an attention line, is the salutation singular or plural?
5. Name one advantage of using the subject line in a business letter? What words in the subject line are usually capitalized?
6. What do we mean by the identification line? Where is it usually typed? If the simplified style is used, how is the subject line typed?
7. When, in the enclosure notation, do we indicate the number of enclosures? Is there any difference between writing out the word *Enclosure* or using *Enc.*, one of the abbreviated forms?
8. When is the mailing notation used? Where is it typed?
9. What is the purpose of the carbon copy notation? Where is it typed?
10. Is it necessary to write the word *Postscript*, or its abbreviation, *P.S.*, when a letter has an afterthought? Explain.

11

Below is a list of the different parts of the business letter, and following is a diagram illustrating them.

Identify these different parts in the list with the alphabetical letter to which it applies.

1. Attention line —
2. Body of letter —
3. Complimentary closing —
4. Date —
5. Enclosure notation —
6. Identification line —
7. Inside address —
8. Letterhead —
9. Mailing notation —
10. Personal notation —
11. Postscript —
12. Reference line —
13. Salutation —
14. Signature —
15. Subject line —

(Diagram detailing the different parts of a business letter)

Addressing the Envelope

The address on the envelope should be typed just below the horizontal center and a little to the left of the vertical center. However, this position may be varied for proper balance, depending on the length and number of lines in the address.

The style should be the same as that of the inside address of the letter. The ZIP Code number must appear on the last line of the address, following the *state*. Several spaces should be left between the last letter of the *state* and the first digit of the ZIP Code number.

The return address of envelopes used in business correspondence is usually printed in the upper left-hand corner with the name and address of the sender. If a plain envelope is used, the return address should be single spaced in the upper left hand corner.

If the letter is being sent by other than regular mail, such as *Special Delivery* or *Registered Mail*, these words should be typed in capital letters on the envelope just below and to the left of the stamp. *Airmail* is generally indicated by using a special airmail envelope, or by attaching a sticker to the envelope:

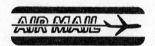

The *Attention Line* and special notation *Care of (c/o)*, should be inserted between the name of the addressee and the address. Notations such as *Personal* and *Confidential* should be placed in the upper left-hand corner directly under the return address. Other special notations such as *Please Forward*, *Hold for Arrival*, etc., should be placed in the lower left-hand corner.

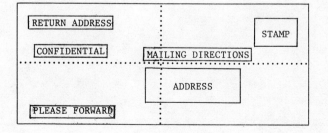

FRED COLLINS
17 East 15th Street
Brooklyn, N.Y. 11218

STAMP

Current Fashions, Inc.
5 West 38 Street
New York, N.Y. 10018

Atlas Chemical Corp.
312 Central Avenue
Newark, NJ 07102

STAMP

CERTIFIED

Personal

Dr. Ruth Ford
17 Elm Street
Austin, TX 78710

NASSAU PHARMACEUTICALS, INC.
5042 Grand Avenue
Camden, N.J. 08101

STAMP

SPECIAL DELIVERY

Research Associates, Inc.
Attention: Dr. B. Burner
843 Constitution Avenue
Niagara Falls, N.Y. 14302

JAMES C. KING
215 Oak Road
Tampa, FL 33602

STAMP

Miss Helen Jackson
27 Baker Court, Apt. 4F
Gary, IN 46401

1. Draw a rectangle measuring 4⅛ by 9½ inches to represent a large commercial No. 10 envelope. Using this rectangle as an envelope, address one for each of the following on the basis of the data given:

    a. Mr. Richard Weber, 23 Ocean Drive, Chicago, Illinois, ZIP Code number 60607.

    b. Purchasing Agent, Franklin Canning Company, 7023 West End Avenue, Seattle, Washington, ZIP Code number 98101.

    c. Mr. Donald Armstrong, Vice-President, American Export Corporation, 364 Main Street, Philadelphia, Pennsylvania, ZIP Code number 19103, special delivery.

    d. Northern Express Corporation, 1234 Hawthorne Drive, Racine, Wisconsin, ZIP Code number 53402, attention of Mr. Joseph E. Barrett, airmail.

    e. Dr. Charles V. Rockwell, Director of Rehabilitation, North Side Medical Center, 1163 Broadway, Brockton, Massachusetts, ZIP Code number 53402, attention of Mr. Joseph E. Barrett, airmail.

2. Draw a rectangle measuring 3⅝ by 6½ inches to represent the small commercial envelope No. 6¾. Using this rectangle as an envelope, address one for each of the following on the basis of the data given:

    a. Ms. Gladys Dean, 21 Sunset Drive, Santa Barbara, California, ZIP Code number 93102.

    b. Dr. Francis Becker, c/o Chairman, Department of Chemistry, State University, Elmira, New York, ZIP Code number 14902.

    c. Miss Elizabeth Nichols, Hotel Riverside Tower, 28 East 31 Street, New York, New York, ZIP Code number 10016, please hold for arrival.

    d. Mr. Theodore Hollenbeck, Director of Research and Development, National Scientific Corporation, 1043 Georgetown Boulevard, Minneapolis, Minnesota, ZIP Code number 55412, confidential, special delivery.

    e. Professor George Karsen, Department of Romance Languages, University of Rochester, Rochester, New York, ZIP Code number 14620, please forward.

    f. Dr. Paul H. Ehrlich, 265 Blackstone Boulevard, Providence, Rhode Island, ZIP Code number 02906, Apartment No. 606.

How to Complain Effectively

What should you do when the new VCR will run only in reverse, your refrigerator freezes the lettuce but melts the ice cream or that new blouse labeled machine-washable shrinks? You need to complain properly—without feeling intimidated or making threats—in order to get results. A bit of preparation and a measure of persistence will help you achieve a satisfactory solution. Follow these guidelines:

Step #1. Organize your records. Be sure that you have these details written down:
- the purchase date and location;
- any verbal guarantees made at the time of purchase;
- model and serial numbers, size, color and brand name of the product. Your file should include all written records, such as a warranty, guarantee, contract, sales and delivery receipts and canceled checks.

Also think through what specific action will remedy the situation: a repair, a refund or a replacement.

Step #2. Contact the business that sold you the merchandise. If you ordered the item by mail or by phone, it's best to put your complaint into writing, being sure to include copies of all pertinent documentation. In your letter, describe in as much detail as possible the specific product defect, and clearly state the solution you desire.

In the case of merchandise purchased from a local store, return to the store in person, taking the merchandise along if possible. Make sure you speak with the appropriate person: If a clerk can't handle the matter, ask to speak with a supervisor, then the store manager. If the store has a complaint or return department, that should be your first stop.

Step #3. What if your letter of complaint hasn't won the desired solution or if store personnel do not offer a satisfactory settlement? You should proceed to the next level of authority: the product's manufacturer. (If you don't have the address, your local librarian can guide you to reference sources.)

Send a letter and copies of your support materials to the manufacturer by registered mail, return receipt requested. (No matter how small the faulty item, it's best not to enclose it until it's requested.) Address your letter to the company president; it will probably be passed along to the consumer-relations department but will have more impact if it's handed down from the head of the company. You may also want to send a copy of your letter to the manufacturer's trade association, but be sure to mention that you

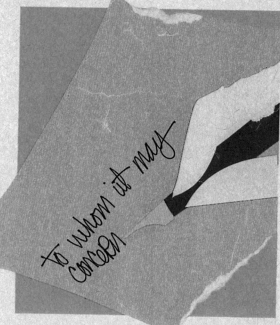

are doing so in the letter itself. Keep copies of all correspondence.

Step #4. If this route doesn't solve the problem, contact your state's consumer-protection agency and your local Better Business Bureau. Most consumer-protection agencies, which are usually part of the attorney general's office, will investigate and mediate consumer disputes. (Your librarian can help you locate the address.) Your Better Business Bureau, a nonprofit organization, keeps a record of consumer complaints and can also help resolve problems.

In both cases, write to the agency, explaining what steps you have already taken and what, if anything, the store or manufacturer has done in response. Send copies of letters you write to these agencies to the store and manufacturer to remind them that you do not intend to let the matter drop until a satisfactory agreement is reached.

—*George L. Beiswinger*

"When Will My Savings Double?"

If you want to figure out how long it will take for money you've invested to double, use the "Rule of 72": Simply divide the number 72 by your interest rate. At a 5 percent rate, for instance, your money will double in about 14 years. A mutual fund that regularly delivers 12 percent interest might dou-

ble your money in just six years!

But don't forget another rule: Generally, the higher the projected rate of return, the greater the risk of losing your principal. And also remember that inflation will play a role in determining the real value of your investment when it comes due. —*Ann Arnott*

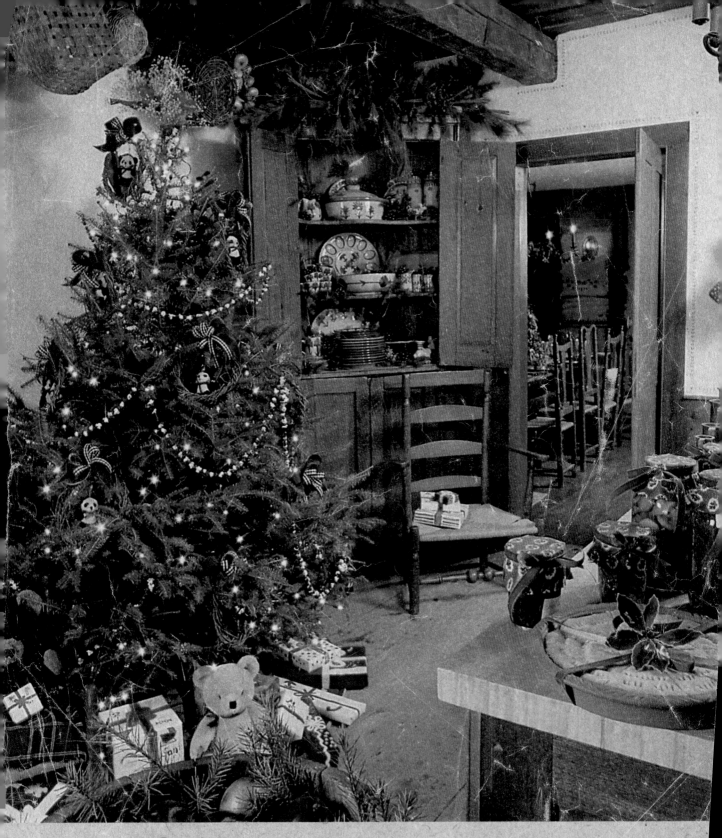

Our holiday house tour ends with the warmth of a traditional country kitchen. Yet another tree is decked with garlands of popcorn and cranberries and mini grapevine wreaths with cheerful ribbon bows. The crowning touch: a bouquet of baby's breath. Other down-home decorations: shiny red apples nestled in deep-green pine needles, just waiting to be savored; baskets, baskets and more baskets; calico-topped, ribbon-tied jars of homemade preserves and boughs of pine.

Folding and Inserting the Letter

For the *standard, letter-size sheet (8½″ by 11″) in the large commercial No. 10 envelope (4⅛″ by 9½″):*
1. Fold the lower third of the sheet up over the message.
2. Fold the upper third of the sheet down.
3. Insert the upper folded edge in the envelope first.

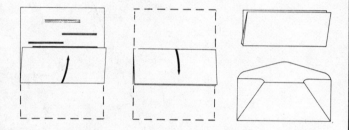

For the *standard, letter-size sheet (8½″ by 11″) in the small commercial No. 6¾ envelope (3⅝″ by 6½″):*
1. Fold the sheet up from the bottom to about one-half inch from the top edge.
2. Fold the right third over.
3. Fold the left third over.
4. Insert the left-folded edge in the envelope first.

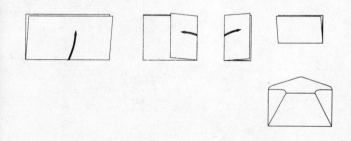

For the *half sheet (5½″ by 8½″) in the small commercial No. 6¾ envelope (3⅝″ by 6½″):*
1. Fold the right third over the message.
2. Fold the left third over.
3. Insert the left folded edge in the envelope first.

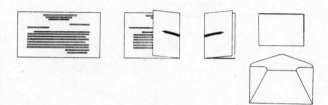

For the *Monarch or Executive size sheet (7¼″ x 10½″) in the No. 7 envelope (3⅞″ by 7½″):*
1. Fold the lower third of the sheet up over the message.
2. Fold the upper third of the sheet down.
3. Insert the upper folded edge in the envelope first.

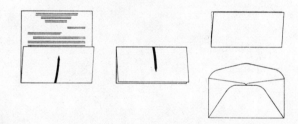

For the *standard, letter-size sheet (8½″ by 11″) in the large commercial window or open panel envelope (4⅛″ by 9½″):*
1. Fold the top third back so that the inside address is positioned properly.
2. Fold the bottom third forward.
3. Insert the folded sheet in such manner that the inside address is visible under the transparent window.

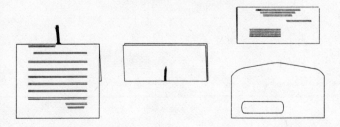

For the *message-reply form (8½" by 7¾") in the large commercial (No. 10) window or open panel envelope (4⅛" by 9½").*

1. Fold the upper half of the topsheet, carbon and pink copy back so that the inside address is positioned properly.
2. Insert the folded sheets in such manner that the inside address is visible under the transparent window.

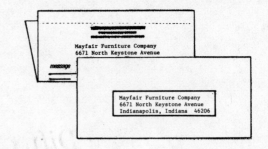

The Different Kinds of
Business Letters

Whether a business is large or small, it receives and writes letters all the time. In fact, while modern business relies very much on the telephone, telegraph and other electronic means of communication, the letter remains one of the most useful tools for handling business transactions.

Because modern business is so complex today, it requires many different kinds of letters. Some of these letters depend on the nature of the business. There are, however, certain kinds of letters that apply to all businesses. These letters have to do with buying and selling, with receiving and collecting payments, with credit, with references, with employment, with the furtherance of good will and with some of the semi-social aspects of business.

In this section we will deal with most of the more frequently used kinds of letters. They will serve as examples of how business letters are written, and what they are intended to do.

LETTERS OF GENERAL INQUIRY

The letter requesting a favor

The letter requesting a favor should be clear, concise and courteous. Begin your letter by stating what you want and why you want it. Then ask for the favor and give additional facts to clarify what you want. End your letter with an expression of appreciation. Be sure your request is reasonable; that is, one that will not mean too much trouble and effort for the person you are writing to. Enclose a stamp or a stamped, self-addressed envelope for the convenience of the person replying.

The letter answering a request for a favor

The answer to such a letter should be prompt and if possible the favor should be granted. The letter can begin by expressing pleasure in being able to help the person who asked the favor. Then follow with the information requested and any helpful suggestions that may be pertinent, and end with an expression of good will.

If it is not possible to grant the favor, it is just as important to be prompt and courteous in replying. Express pleasure at receiving the request. Give your reason for your inability to grant the favor. If you can, suggest other likely sources of information and conclude with an expression of good will.

Examples of such letters follow.

202 College Avenue
Dayton, Ohio 45401
October 26, 19__

American Hospital Association
1381 East 60 Street
Chicago, Illinois 60637

Gentlemen:

In connection with my school work at the University of Dayton, I am engaged in a research project on "A Survey of Salaries Paid to Laboratory Personnel in Hospitals."

Please send me any data, pamphlets or other information that you may have on this subject. Any suggestions you may have to offer will be appreciated.

I shall be grateful for your cooperation in this research project. If you wish, I shall be happy to send you a copy of my report when it is completed.

Yours very truly,

Walter Spencer

Walter Spencer

(Letter requesting a favor)

AMERICAN HOSPITAL ASSOCIATION
1381 East 60 Street
Chicago, Illinois 60637

October 30, 19__

Mr. Walter Spencer
202 College Avenue
Dayton, Ohio 45401

Dear Mr. Spencer:

Your letter of October 26 requesting information on salaries paid to laboratory personnel in hospitals reached me yesterday afternoon.

I am enclosing a copy of our most recent report on salaries paid to hospital personnel. The data listed on pages 10 and 11 should be particularly helpful.

For more detailed and current information, I suggest that you write to the U.S. Department of Labor, Washington, D.C. 20025. This government agency makes thorough salary studies of the different occupational groups. It is noted for its excellent, up-to-date reports.

I will be happy to receive a copy of your completed report.

Cordially yours,

Edward Larson

Edward Larson
Secretary

EL:al
Enc.

(Letter granting a favor)

AMERICAN HOSPITAL ASSOCIATION
1381 East 60 Street
Chicago, Illinois 60637

October 30, 19__

Mr. Walter Spencer
202 College Avenue
Dayton, Ohio 45401

Dear Mr. Spencer:

Thank you for your letter of October 26 requesting information on salaries paid to laboratory personnel in hospitals.

We do not have recent salary data on laboratory positions; accordingly, we cannot furnish you the information you need in connection with your research project.

I suggest that you write to the U.S. Department of Labor, Washington, D.C. 20025 for detailed and up-to-date salary data on the national level. Our own Department of Labor at Springfield has such data available for hospital laboratory positions within the state. Both governmental agencies are noted for their thorough salary studies, as well as their reliable reports.

Please accept our best wishes for success in your research project.

Sincerely yours,

Edward Larson

Edward Larson
Secretary

EL:al

(Letter expressing inability to grant a favor)

TOWER STATIONERY COMPANY
1403 Charles Street
Binghamton, N.Y. 13902

April 10, 19__

Mr. Walter Kane
The Parkever Pen Corporation
1148 West End Avenue
Rochester, N.Y. 14603

Dear Mr. Kane:

Do you manufacture pens that can be used with cartridges and also as conventional pens? My sales personnel inform me that here have been many requests for such pens these past few days.

If such pens are available, please send me a brochure describing such pens, as well as the price list. Can shipment be made within ten days after receipt of order?

A prompt reply will be appreciated.

Sincerely yours,

William Sullivan
William Sullivan
Purchasing Agent

WS:al

(Letter of inquiry from a possible buyer)

The letter of inquiry regarding a possible purchase

This type of letter is written by someone who is considering the purchase of a product or service. The letter must be clear and must specify what is needed. Begin by stating what you want. Then ask for whatever information you need to help you in deciding whether or not you will buy. You may wish to describe the product and how it works; you may want to know service requirements, price, terms, delivery time, guarantee, etc. Since this kind of letter is of a strictly business nature, do not enclose a stamp or a stamped, self-addressed envelope.

THE PARKEVER PEN CORPORATION
1148 West End Avenue   Rochester, N.Y. 14603

April 12, 19__

Mr. William Sullivan
Purchasing Agent
Tower Stationery Company
1403 Charles Street
Binghamton, N.Y. 13902

Dear Mr. Sullivan:

I am happy to inform you that we have a complete line of pens that can be used with cartridges or converted readily for use in the conventional manner. Judging from orders received, it appears that these pens are increasing in popularity.

A brochure showing the various pen styles is enclosed. The Princess and Vassar styles are "best sellers."

As to color and point size, there is quite a selection. We have them in four colors--blue, green, black and silver. The penpoints come in three sizes--fine, medium and broad.

A price list is enclosed in the brochure. Trade discounts depend on the size of the order. Regarding delivery, we can make shipment within four work days from the date of your order.

Our district representative, Mr. Arthur Martin, will be in Binghamton on the 14th of April. He can show you our full line and supply any additional information regarding our products. He will call you in the morning and arrange to see you at your convenience.

Please let me know if we can be of further assistance.

Sincerely yours,

Walter Kane
Walter Kane
Regional Sales Manager

WK:al
Encl.

(Answer to letter of inquiry from a possible buyer)

Suggested answers to a possible buyer

1. If you are able to supply what the writer of the letter wants, then your reply should really be a sales letter; that is, it should be written with the idea of convincing the prospective customer that he should buy your product or the service you offer. Begin your answer by expressing your pleasure at being able to supply what he wants. Then bring out the best points of what you offer and supply the information requested, together with any additional information that will help to make the sale. Conclude by expressing your willingness and ability to be of further service.

2. If you cannot supply the product or the service, you might offer an alternate solution. Begin your letter by acknowledging receipt of the inquiry. Then explain why you cannot supply what is wanted. Then, not only suggest, but describe your alternate suggestion. End your letter with an expression of good will and offer to be of further assistance. Though this is a negative letter, it is also a sales letter in that you have made an alternate suggestion.

THE PARKEVER PEN CORPORATION
1148 West End Avenue   Rochester, N.Y. 14603

April 12, 19__

Mr. William Sullivan
Purchasing Agent
Tower Stationery Company
1403 Charles Street
Binghamton, N.Y. 13902

Dear Mr. Sullivan:

Thank you for writing to us about a type of pen for which you have received many recent requests.

We do not carry such pens. However, I would suggest our new COSMOS pen with giant cartridge. Although just recently introduced, it is a "best seller" and is increasing in popularity, judging from orders received.

Our COSMOS pen, because of the large capacity of the giant cartridge, requires infrequent replacement of the cartridge and has won acceptance of many conventional pen owners. The variety of ink colors available and the low cost of replacement cartridges are additional desirable features.

A descriptive folder highlighting the many features of this pen is enclosed. The price list appears on the last page. Regarding delivery, we can make shipment within four work days from the date of your order.

Our district representative, Mr. Arthur Martin, will be in Binghamton on the 14th of April. He can show you our full line and supply any additional information regarding our products. He will call you in the morning and arrange to see you at your convenience.

Do let me know if we can be of further assistance.

Sincerely yours,

Walter Kane

Walter Kane
Regional Sales Manager

WK:al
Enc.

(Acknowledgement of letter from possible buyer, with alternate suggestion)

(A — Making a request)

1. In connection with a course at a local college, you are making a survey of the reading habits of the American public. Write a letter to the book editor of a national weekly requesting assistance in this project.

2. As manager of a commercial establishment, you are planning to purchase a variety of office machines in connection with a contemplated expansion of the accounting section. Write a letter to one of the larger office machine dealers in your community requesting catalogs and other pertinent information.

3. Assume that you have misplaced the driver's manual which you received when you first took possession of your automobile. It is essential that another manual be obtained for reference purposes. Write a letter to the automobile manufacturer requesting that another driver's manual be sent to you.

4. Write to one of the major oil companies requesting travel information for a one-month, cross-country, motor trip you and your family expect to take in the near future. Indicate in your letter when you will start the trip, the places you wish to visit, side trips you would like to make and the return date. Suggest that their recommendations regarding other scenic or historic points to be visited will be appreciated.

5. Assume that you, a production supervisor in a large metal company, are interested in obtaining a paint which is rust, acid and alkali-resistant. This paint is needed for coating pails used in the chemical industry. Write to the American Paint Association stating the problem, requesting their technical assistance, and asking where such paint can be obtained. The association's address is 625 Lacquer Boulevard, Pittsburgh, Pennsylvania, ZIP Code number 15219.

(B — Answering the request)

1. Assume that you are a book editor of a national weekly. You have just received a letter from a college student who is making a survey of the reading habits of the American public. The student has asked for your help in this survey. Reply that you are not in a position to help in this survey because you do not have sufficient data on the subject.

2. Assume that you are a director of sales for a large office machine company. You have received a letter from the manager of an out-of-state firm. The manager states that they are planning to purchase a variety of office machines in connection with the expansion of their accounting section and asks for catalogs and other pertinent information. Prepare a reply advising that the latest catalogs and other technical information can be obtained from the district distributor to whom you are forwarding the manager's letter.

3. Assume that you are a director of public relations for a large automobile manufacturing company. A letter received from an automobile owner requests another driver's manual to replace the one he has lost. There is no driver's manual available for his model of automobile. However, you still have a small supply of booklets containing descriptive material as well as technical information for this particular model. Prepare an appropriate reply.

4. Assume that you are a travel consultant with a major oil company. A request has been received for travel information in connection with a contemplated one-month, cross-country motor trip. The person making the request names several places he intends to visit and side trips he expects to take. He also asks for your recommendations regarding scenic or historic points to visit. Prepare a reply stating that a travel kit containing maps, a guide to points of interest and a directory of recommended hotels, motels and restaurants will be mailed to him in a few days.

5. Assume that you are a technical advisor with the American Paint Association. A letter from a production supervisor of a large metal company has been referred to you for reply. The production supervisor is interested in obtaining a paint which is rust, acid and alkali-resistant and also asks where such a paint may be obtained. You have available a four-page brochure entitled "Paint for Industry" which contains this information. Prepare an appropriate reply.

SALES LETTERS
(including sales promotion)

A business concern is always interested in promoting sales. This can be done through salesmen, newspaper and magazine advertising, circulars, catalogs, booklets, brochures and, of course, letters. There are a number of different kinds of sales letters that a business uses. Among these are:

The letter that does not offer a particular item for sale, but offers the products of the company as a whole, including its special services. This is known as *institutional advertising*. It is intended to create good will by building up the idea that the company makes fine products and renders good service.

The letter that offers a particular item for sale at a special price, sometimes for a limited time.

The letter that announces a new facility, service or item to attract new customers and keep old ones.

The letter that answers an inquiry about a particular item and aims to bring about a sale.

All sales letters must possess these qualities:

They must attract attention.

They must arouse interest and stimulate a desire to buy.

They must be convincing about the product(s) offered.

They must inspire the reader to act by deciding to buy without delay.

To arouse interest a letter may use questions, catch phrases, proverbs, humorous statements, cartoons, novel headlines, unusual thoughts, unexpected commands and similar devices. Below are a few examples of attention-getting opening lines used in sales promotion letters:

Are you anxious to reduce your heat bills this winter?

School opens in only four more weeks! Buy . . .

Our storewide sale begins today! Don't wait!

Your neighbor is one of our satisfied customers. Why not you?

Are you as popular as you would like to be?

Tell it to the Marines? No, but you should know that . . .

There is no fuel like an old fuel! Use coal for greater . . .

Pep up your car engine! Get more miles to the gallon! Switch to BRAND gasoline now!

Come in and browse through our remodeled 7th and 8th floors. They're chock-full of brand-new furniture at bargain prices.

All infants, toddlers and teen-age wear now on sale! Come and get it!

A sales letter should also appeal to any one or more of the following basic human desires:

(1) personal ambition
(2) the desire to protect the family
(3) personal health and safety
(4) making money
(5) pride of possession
(6) attracting the opposite sex
(7) saving time or money
(8) personal popularity
(9) the desire to be stylish
(10) the desire to emulate other people
(11) comfort and pleasure
(12) leisure
(13) social approval
(14) education
(15) children's success
(16) making friends
(17) having a nice home
(18) belonging to a club or society
(19) being considered up to date
(20) pride in accomplishment
(21) exercising one's talent
(22) being respected in the community
(23) being well-dressed
(24) being able to travel
— and a host of other human desires.

Sometimes a good sales letter can use testimonials from other satisfied customers, offer guarantees, present the results of tests, or describe the business concern offering the products.

The final paragraph in a sales letter should motivate to action. The prospective buyer must be encouraged to act immediately. A business reply card, a simple order form, or a postage-free return envelope are some of the ways to encourage prompt action by mail. Following are some examples of effective closing paragraphs for sales letters:

For a generous sample, mail the enclosed postage-free card to us.

For additional information, send us the enclosed card with your name and address.

Our representative will be glad to drop in to see you within the next few days, if you will just mail the enclosed postcard back to us with your name and address.

Let us demonstrate our Wilson Vacuum Cleaner in your own home. Call 566-6200 for an appointment.

Your name and address on enclosed form will bring you *Our World Today* for a two-months trial period. Or, if you want to subscribe for a year, send check or money order for $5.95. If, after you've received four issues, you don't like the magazine and wish to cancel your subscription, let us know and we'll refund your money.

A great many business firms answer sales inquiries about their products or services with specially prepared printed forms. These printed forms either give as much of the information requested as possible, or are mailed with a catalog, a brochure or other piece of advertising that contains information.

Samples of the different types of sales letters and a printed form follow:

ROYAL McBEE CORPORATION

850 THIRD AVENUE ◆ NEW YORK, N.Y. 10022

July 27, 19__

Mr. ////////////
Purchasing Agent
///////////////////
//////////////////
//////////////////

Dear Mr. //////////:

Thank you for your recent request for information on the new FILETAPE
ROYALTYPER. It is a pleasure to send the enclosed material and we hope
that you will find the information helpful.

This automatic typing unit presents a low cost system for fast, reliable
production of office documents, forms, and personalized correspondence
which contain portions of repetitive information. Purchase orders, invoices, production orders, legal documents and unlimited paragraph selection
for correspondence are but a few of the many time and money saving
applications.

I hope you will permit us to demonstrate the Filetape Royaltyper to your
organization as soon as possible. We believe that it is truly the most
versatile automatic typing system on the market and I think further investigation on your part will convince you of this.

We appreciate the interest you have shown in this new product and our
Company. If we can be of service to you in anyway, please contact us
at your earliest convenience.

Very truly yours,

David W. Florence

David W. Florence
Sales Manager
Automated Equipment

DWF:al
Enclosure

P.S. In addition to the purchase and rental plans, the Filetape Royaltyper
      is also available at an extremely low cost lease plan.

(Sales promotion letter in regard to a particular item)

DOW'S DEPARTMENT STORE
1300 P STREET
LINCOLN, NEBRASKA 68501

Paul Goodwin
Vice - President

September 20, 19__

Mr. Harold Cooper
1063 12 Street
Lincoln, Nebraska 68502

Dear Mr. Cooper:

Welcome to Lincoln!

Dow's Department Store is happy to greet you and your family--newcomers to
our community. We are glad that you have decided to make your new
home with us. We know that you are going to like it here.

Ours is one of the largest department stores in Nebraska--especially equipped
to serve the home owner. Whether it be furniture, clothing, household
furnishings and supplies, paint, tools, garden supplies and equipment,
stationery,..., we have it if you need it. During the years, Dow's has
earned the reputation of selling the best brand products at very reasonable prices.

You may find it very convenient to open a charge account with us. Let us talk
it over when you are in our store. We are open until 9 p.m. on Tuesdays
and Thursdays; on other store nights we are open until 6 p.m. There is
plenty of free parking available in our parking lot.

Won't you and your family visit us soon? We'll be happy to meet you and show
you around. Please bring this letter with you and receive a gift from us,
a token of our hospitality and well wishes.

Cordially yours,

Paul Goodwin

Paul Goodwin

(Sales promotion letter — institutional)

25

ROYAL McBEE CORPORATION
850 Third Avenue ◆ New York, N.Y. 10022

/////////////////////

/////////////
/////////////
/////////////

/////////////

    Thank you for your interest in Royal McBee and
its business machines.

    I am pleased to enclose the literature which you
requested. I trust that this information will suit
your needs.

    If I can be of further assistance, please feel
free to call upon me.

                 Cordially yours,

                 Richard J. Cannon
                 Public Relations Adminstrator

RJC:al

Enclosure

(Sales promotion letter answering a letter of general inquiry)

ATLANTIC MACHINE COMPANY
Chester, Pennsylvania 19017

Here is the material you requested recently. We hope it
contains the information you
need. If you would like to
know more about our machines
or how they may be used by
your firm, mail the postpaid
card enclosed in the booklet.
We will send you a prompt reply or, if you wish, will have
our representative call at any
time convenient to you.

Thank you for your interest.

        Sincerely yours,

        John Watson
        Executive Director

(Printed form of answer to general sales inquiry)

PRACTICE EXERCISES

1. Assume that you are a sales manager for a large retail clothing establishment. A private sale for regular customers is to be held prior to its public announcement in the newspapers. Prepare a suitable sales promotion letter.

2. Assume that you are the owner of a summer resort. You wish to maintain friendly contact with your former guests. Prepare a letter expressing the hope that you may be their host again next summer. Mention the innovations and improvements that have been made for the greater comfort and pleasure of the guests and suggest the need for early reservations.

3. In connection with the forthcoming opening of an automobile service station in your community, you have been asked to prepare a sales promotion letter. Include the following in your letter: nationally known brands of the items offered in the service station for all types of automobiles, modern equipment, specially-trained personnel, reasonable prices, opening date, hours of service, souvenirs during opening week and the desire to render the best service to the car owners of the community.

4. Write a suitable sales letter to be sent to home owners urging them to subscribe to *House and Home*, a monthly magazine devoted to home decoration, maintenance and improvement.

5. Assume that you are director of a children's summer camp located 50 miles from the city where you live. Prepare a suitable letter to be sent to parents suggesting that they enroll their children as campers for the approaching summer. Include in the letter the following and any other information that would be of particular interest to parents of young children: athletic and recreational facilities, educational and social programs, sleeping accommodations, food standards and facilities, counselors, nursing staff, rates and enrollment procedure.

LETTERS REGARDING CREDIT AND CREDIT STANDING

Credit is a very important part of our economy. When a business renders a bill to a customer for merchandise bought or services rendered; when a bank lends money to a depositor; when an individual buys something on the installment plan— we say that these are transactions on credit. Credit is really an expression of faith in ability to pay for merchandise bought or services rendered or money advanced.

An individual asking for credit is generally required to furnish information about income, employment, personal property, real estate holdings, marital and family status and bank references.

Business firms seeking credit are required to furnish financial statements and bank and trade references. Other sources of credit information are credit agencies such as Dun and Bradstreet and trade associations.

Many credit transactions are handled by means of letters and some are handled by printed forms.

Letters regarding *business credit standing* fall into the following categories:

(1) Correspondence between two business firms about a third business firm that has asked for credit

(2) Correspondence between two business firms in regard to a request for credit from one to another

Correspondence regarding credit standing among business firms is usually with banks, trade and credit agencies and other business firms. Often a firm asking for credit is required to submit a financial statement which serves as one of the bases for consideration of credit.

Correspondence regarding credit standing of an individual usually involves landlords, savings banks, local credit bureaus, business firms that may have dealt with individuals, employers, and individuals whose names have been given as credit references.

Whether the correspondence concerns a business firm or an individual, it should at all times be frank, factual and sincere. It can be assumed that all credit correspondence is held confidential. To save time and extra work, many firms use form letters or printed forms to elicit information or grant or refuse credit. Some business firms prefer the telephone as the quickest and most efficient way of handling credit information.

The letter (or form) granting credit to another firm or to an individual should be both a "welcome" and a "sales" letter. It should always be friendly and courteous and should contain the following, along with such additional information as particular circumstances require:

(1) A statement to the effect that the credit has been granted

(2) Where an order was part of the request for credit, the letter should state that the order is being filled — on open invoice

(3) A statement of the terms and conditions under which credit has been granted

(4) A statement describing the services and merchandise that are available to the new credit customer

(5) An expression of appreciation of the opportunity to be of service

(6) An expression of hope that business relations in the future will continue to be cordial and mutually advantageous

The letter (or form) refusing credit is not easy to write. It requires tact and care in wording. Yet, a refusal can also be friendly, courteous and cordial, to retain good will. Here are some of the points a letter of refusal should include:

(1) Though the credit is refused on the basis of credit information received, assure the reader that the refusal need not be permanent.

(2) Credit may be reconsidered in the future if conditions or additional information warrant a more favorable decision.

(3) It is advisable to suggest to the rejected applicant that doing business on a cash basis has certain advantages, such as a discount for cash and speedier attention to orders.

(4) A letter rejecting an application for credit from an individual should minimize or even omit any reference to ineligibility for credit. Instead, the advantages of buying for cash should be brought out.

(5) A credit refusal to a business firm should, on the other hand, deal frankly with the reasons for denying the credit.

(6) A refusal letter should end with the suggestion that reapplication can be made at some future time when the adverse credit rating has been corrected, and with a cordial expression of appreciation.

Following are a variety of letters relating to credit and credit standing.

Letter from an individual requesting credit

Such a letter must begin by stating its purpose and it must offer to furnish references or supply other needed information.

```
                                       88 Cleveland Avenue South
                                       St. Paul, Minnesota  55101
                                       September 18, 19__


Coleman's Department Store
9403 Bush Avenue
St. Paul, Minnesota  55106

Gentlemen:

     I wish to open a credit account with your department
store.

     If there are references or other information required,
please let me know.

                                       Very truly yours,

                                       Doris Lindsay

                                       Doris Lindsay
                                       (Mrs. Richard E. Lindsay)
```

(Letter from an individual requesting credit)

27

Letter acknowledging credit request from an individual

Sometimes a request for credit does not give enough information that will enable a firm to evaluate the credit standing of an individual. The letter acknowledging such a request should ask for additional information, and should explain why it is needed. Often the acknowledging letter is accompanied by a printed credit application form for the customer to fill out. The letter should be friendly in tone and sincere in manner. It should end by suggesting a prompt reply.

Letter granting credit to an individual

This type of letter should be warm and cordial. All the necessary information regarding the credit that has been granted should be given in the letter, including the terms of payment for purchases made. The letter should end on a note of assurance that the customer will receive prompt and courteous service and express appreciation of the opportunity to render service.

Letter refusing credit to an individual

A letter of refusal has to be very carefully worded so that the recipient will not be offended. Such a letter should give a good reason for the refusal and at the same time offer a possibility for reconsidering the request for credit at some future time. The letter should mention the fine service and excellent merchandise that is available to the customer on a cash basis and the special sales that enable the customer to save money.

COLEMAN'S DEPARTMENT STORE
9403 Bush Avenue
St. Paul, Minnesota 55106

September 21, 19__

Mrs. Doris Lindsay
88 Cleveland Avenue South
St. Paul, Minn. 55101

Dear Mrs. Lindsay:

Thank you for your letter of September 18 expressing an interest in opening a charge account with us.

To enable us to open a charge account for you with a minimum of delay, please fill in the information requested on the enclosed card and return it promptly in the addressed, stamped envelope.

We look forward to the pleasure of adding your name to our growing list of charge customers.

Yours sincerely,

Martin Hunt
Martin Hunt
Credit Manager

Enc.

(Letter acknowledging credit request from an individual)

COLEMAN'S DEPARTMENT STORE
9403 Bush Avenue
St. Paul, Minnesota 55106

October 26, 19__

Mrs. Doris Lindsay
88 Cleveland Avenue South
St. Paul, Minn. 55101

Dear Mrs. Lindsay:

We are happy to inform you that your request has been granted and a charge account has been opened in your name.

An identification plate with your name, address and account number is enclosed. The booklet explains how the plate is to be used and also tells you about the many services this store offers for your convenience.

We hope you will enjoy your visits to our store. However, you may find it convenient to order by telephone. Such orders will receive our usual prompt and courteous attention.

It is our desire that you remain a satisfied customer for many years. We appreciate the opportunity of being of service.

Sincerely yours,

Martin Hunt
Martin Hunt
Credit Manager

MH:al
Encl.

(Letter granting credit to an individual)

THE CAPITAL DEPARTMENT STORE
204 East Washington Avenue • Madison, Wisconsin 53703

November 27, 19__

Mrs. Jean Hull
486 Oak Place
Madison, Wisconsin 53702

Dear Mrs. Hull:

We appreciate your recent inquiry about credit accommodations.

The information given on the credit application is not sufficient to enable us to open a charge account for you at the present time. If, in the future, you feel that there is additional information which you would want us to consider, please visit Mr. Robert Kern in our credit department. He will be glad to confer with you.

In the meantime, we hope that you will continue as a cash customer at Capital. Our quality merchandise at reasonable prices, our telephone and daily delivery services, our free parking and other customer services--these are some of the reasons why so many find shopping at the Capital Department Store convenient and desirable.

May we remind you of our special weekly sales advertised each Friday in the local newspapers. You will realize considerable savings on these specially priced articles.

Sincerely yours,

Larry Webb
Larry Webb
Credit Manager

LW:al

(Letter refusing credit to an individual)

Letter from a firm that has just bought a business and asks for a continuance of credit previously given

This is a letter that expresses confidence. Not only does it convey the idea that the business is profitable, but it states that it has been bought by the previous owner's manager who knows its operation. It also gives a number of very good references. The writer of this letter feels sure that the credit he asks for will be granted.

SOUTH SIDE ATHLETIC SUPPLIES
380 South 14 Street
Grand Rapids, Michigan 49501

October 15, 19__

American Athletic Equipment Company
821 Diamond Avenue
Flint, Michigan 48502

Gentlemen:

I have recently purchased this athletic supply store from Mr. Bernard Stone and wish to continue the open account with your company enjoyed by my predecessor.

I had been Mr. Stone's store manager for the past six years and have just taken over the business since Mr. Stone's departure to Colorado for health reasons.

The following is a list of references. Feel free to communicate with them for credit information.

First National Bank, 2142 Broad Street, Grand Rapids, Michigan 49502.

Miller Reality Corporation, 421 East Fourth Street, Grand Rapids, Michigan 49502.

Mr. Arthur P. Meyers, Athletic Director, Michigan Community College, 375 Court Street, Grand Rapids, Michigan 49503.

Mr. Thomas Walsh, President, Retail Merchants Association, 384 Broad Street, Grand Rapids, Michigan 49501.

I am enclosing an order for athletic equipment. I hope that you will be able to make prompt shipment.

Very truly yours,

Martin Burke

Martin Burke
Proprietor

MB:al
Encl.

REVERE MUSICAL SUPPLIES, Inc.
831 Symphony Avenue
Charleston, W. Va. 25304

January 26, 19__

Electronic Phonograph Company
8306 West Main Street
Portsmouth, Va. 23705

Gentlemen:

Please ship by express on open account the following as listed in your current trade catalogue:

12 portable electric phonographs, model 1409, at $39.90 each.
4 califones, model 12W-9, at $103.50 each.

Very truly yours,

Ralph Brooks

Ralph Brooks
Purchasing Agent

RB:AL

(Letter placing an order on open account)

Letters regarding orders to be sent on open account

The four letters that follow have to do with (1) an order to be shipped on credit or open account; (2) the acknowledgment of the order by the firm receiving it, requesting credit information; (3) the final letter to the customer advising that credit has been granted and shipment of the order made; and (4) the final letter to a business firm advising that credit has not been granted.

These letters, while entirely business-like, are cordial in tone and confident in manner. They express a desire to do business together.

ELECTRONIC PHONOGRAPH COMPANY
8306 WEST MAIN STREET
PORTSMOUTH, VIRGINIA 23705

February 2, 19__

Mr. Ralph Brooks
Purchasing Agent
Revere Musical Supplies, Inc.
831 Symphony Avenue
Charleston, W. Va. 25304

Dear Mr. Brooks:

Thank you for your order of January 26 for 12 portable electric phonographs and 4 califones.

Since this is your first order with us, we must ask you to complete the enclosed credit application form and attach a copy of your latest financial statement. Of course, this information will be held in strict confidence.

Upon receipt of the application blank and financial statement, we will give your credit request prompt and careful attention.

In the meantime, we have set aside the items you have ordered and will ship them as soon as your credit rating is approved.

We look forward to the opportunity of serving you.

Sincerely yours,

Ralph G. Allen

Ralph G. Allen
Sales Manager

RGA:AL
ENC.

(Letter acknowledging firm's request for credit)

ELECTRONIC PHONOGRAPH COMPANY
8306 WEST MAIN STREET
PORTSMOUTH, VIRGINIA 23705

February 10, 19__

Mr. Ralph Brooks
Purchasing Agent
Revere Musical Supplies, Inc.
831 Symphony Avenue
Charleston, W.Va. 25304

Dear Mr. Brooks:

The 12 portable electric phonographs and 4 califones that you ordered
on January 26 are being shipped by express to you today. The terms
are 2/10, net 30.

Your application for credit was favorably considered and we are happy
to welcome you as a new account. You will be allowed as much as $1,200
worth of merchandise on credit.

As one of our accounts, you will receive display posters and other sales
promotion material from us. Our salesmen are available to discuss with
you how our products may be used to a greater degree in your merchandizing
efforts.

We hope that this order will be the beginning of a long and pleasant
relationship with you.

                                        Sincerely yours,

                                        Ralph G. Allen

                                        Ralph G. Allen
                                        Sales Manager

RGA:al

(Letter granting firm's request for credit)

Letters regarding credit standing

There are two kinds of answers to inquiries regarding credit standing: those that are favorable and those that are unfavorable.

Letters that give favorable credit information can be frank, factual and sincere. Very often a favorable credit report includes a recommendation regarding the firm or individual who is the subject of the report.

Letters that are unfavorable as to credit standing must be written with great discretion. Very often, in the exercise of such discretion, a letter answering an inquiry as to credit standing will not even mention the name of the applicant. Many firms who find it necessary to give an unfavorable report prefer to do so over the telephone, rather than commit themselves on paper in the form of a letter.

NEWPORT MANUFACTURING COMPANY, Inc.
5700 West Douglas Avenue
Des Moines, Iowa 50318

February 1, 19___

First National Bank of Fargo
308 East Main Street
Fargo, North Dakota 58101

Gentlemen:

The Perry Sales Company recently applied for a credit account with our firm. Your bank was given as a reference.

We would appreciate any information regarding the company's ability to meet its financial obligations. Naturally, your reply will be held in strict confidence.

Thank you for your cooperation in this matter.

Very truly yours,

Bruce Lyons
Bruce Lyons
Credit Manager

BL:AL

(Letter requesting credit standing)

The COSMOS Corporation
45 St. Joseph Street • Sioux Falls, S. Dak. 57101

March 14, 19___

Mr. Andrew Nelson
Credit Manager
Southwest Commercial Company
140 West First Street
Reno, Nevada 89501

Dear Mr. Nelson:

It is a pleasure to answer your letter of March 10 regarding Johnson's Appliance Company.

We have had considerable business dealings with this company for the past six years. Our records indicate that Johnson's Appliance Company has always paid its bills promptly. Its credit limit with us has been $2000.

We do not hesitate to recommend that credit be extended to this company.

Sincerely yours,

Ralph Owens
Ralph Owens
Treasurer

RO:un

(Letter from a firm giving a favorable credit reference)

The COSMOS Corporation
45 St. Joseph Street • Sioux Falls, S. Dak. 57101

April 10, 19___

Mr. Sidney Borden
Credit Department
General Chemical Corporation
246 Polymer Circle
Billings, Mont. 59107

Dear Mr. Borden:

We regret to say that the individual about whom you inquired in your letter of April 7 has an unsatisfactory credit record with this company.

He has been our customer for the past three years and we have had great difficulty in collecting from him on several occasions. Recently we were compelled to make collection through our attorney. Future shipments will be made to him only on a cash basis.

It is requested that this information be kept strictly confidential.

Sincerely yours,

Ralph Owens
Ralph Owens
Treasurer

RO:al

(Letter from a firm giving an unfavorable credit reference)

ATLAS MERCANTILE CORPORATION
40 CULVERT STREET
NASHVILLE, TENNESSEE 37202

February 3, 19___

Central Supply Company, Inc.
3130 North May Avenue
Oklahoma City, Oklahoma 73102

Gentlemen:

Thank you for sending us a financial statement in connection with
your recent order and application for credit.

An analysis of your most recent financial figures discloses insuf-
ficient working capital. We will not be able to extend the credit
privilege you requested until this deficiency is remedied. Perhaps
in the future, an improvement in your financial condition will permit us to open a credit account for your company.

Be assured, however, that we are anxious to be of service. If you
wish, we will send the merchandise to you collect. Naturally, you
will be entitled to a two percent cash discount.

Perhaps you would like to reduce the size of your order now and
reorder the balance at a later date.

Please let us know as soon as possible what action to take on your
order. Shipment can be made three days after receipt of your instructions.

We appreciate the opportunity to serve you.

Very truly yours,

John R. Shaw

John R. Shaw
General Manager

JRS:al

(Letter from a business firm refusing credit to another business firm)

1. Write a letter to one of the large department stores in your community stating that you wish to open a credit account. Indicate how long you have resided in the community and the length of time you have been a cash customer.

2. Assume that you are credit manager for a large department store. You have received a letter from a cash customer requesting that a charge account be opened. Prepare a suitable letter acknowledging the request and enclose a credit application form for additional information.

3. You, a credit manager for a large department store, receive a credit application form listing a local bank as one of the references. Write a letter to the bank requesting credit information about the applicant.

4. Assume that you are a bank official in charge of credit referrals. A request for credit information about a depositor has been received. Your records show that this person has maintained a sizable bank balance for many years and has been a satisfactory depositor in all respects. Prepare a suitable reply giving favorable credit information.

5. You, a bank official in charge of credit referrals, have received a request for credit information about a depositor who has frequently overdrawn his account. The records indicate that he is a poor credit risk. Write a letter giving an unfavorable credit rating for this person.

6. You are credit manager for a large department store. Investigation discloses that a cash customer who wishes to open a charge account has a good credit rating. Prepare a suitable letter granting credit to this customer.

7. You, a credit manager for a large department store, have ascertained that a customer who wishes to open a charge account has a poor credit rating. Prepare an appropriate letter refusing credit to this customer.

8. Assume that you are manager for a manufacturing company. An order for $300 worth of goods on a credit basis has been received from a new customer. Prepare an appropriate letter requesting that certain credit information be sent you as soon as possible.

9. As manager for a manufacturing company, write a letter to a trade association requesting credit information about a new customer who recently sent in an order for goods on a credit basis.

10. Assume that you are an official of a trade association. You have received a request for credit information about a business firm you regard as an excellent credit risk. Write an appropriate reply.

11. You, an official of a trade association, have received a request for credit information about a business firm you regard as a very poor credit risk. The firm has been slow in its payments and has on occasion been involved in litigation for failure to pay its debts. Prepare a suitable reply.

12. As manager for a manufacturing company, you have ascertained that the new customer who recently ordered $300 worth of goods on a credit basis has an excellent credit rating. Write a suitable letter granting credit up to $500.

13. You, the manager for a manufacturing company, have ascertained that a new customer who recently ordered a sizable amount of goods on a credit basis is a very poor credit risk. Write that you are unable to extend credit at this time, but that your company can make shipment on a cash basis.

LETTERS REGARDING ORDERS

Orders for merchandise can be placed by telephone, telegram, printed purchase order form or by letter.

A letter ordering merchandise should contain all necessary information. It should be specific, accurate and complete; otherwise, the order may be delayed or misinterpreted. The following information is essential in a letter placing an order:

1. The date.
2. The request, using such expressions as:
    Please ship . . .
    Please send . . .
    Please enter our order for . . .
    We need the following merchandise . . .

3. If a particular method of sending the order is desired, indicate whether it is to be by railway express, air express, air freight, ordinary parcel post, air parcel post, motor freight or local truck or messenger. Also state whether the shipment is to be made c.o.d. (*cash on delivery*) for freight only or for the entire amount of the bill, or *f.o.b.* (free on board) destination or point of shipment. If a shipment is sent f.o.b. point of shipment, it means that the shipping charges will be added to the bill; if a shipment is sent f.o.b. destination, it means that the shipping charges have been absorbed in the amount of the bill.

4. If the point of destination is not the same as the address of the firm or individual placing the order, clearly indicate the destination address.

5. Include in the order the following: (a) quantity desired; (b) unit (each, dozen, pound, ton, copy, etc.); (c) catalog or model number or trade name(type, kind, size, color,

etc.); (d) price; (e) the extension and total amount are optional.

6. Indicate terms and method of payment: time within which payment of the bill will be made; trade or special discount; whether the order is to be sent on a consignment basis or open account, or *c.o.d.* for the amount of the bill and the shipping charges; or whether the order is accompanied by check or money order or currency.

7. Indicate period of time within which the order is desired, or whether it is a "rush" order and must be filled immediately.

8. Signature: An impersonal complimentary closing, such as *Very truly yours*, should precede the signature of the purchaser.

Today, the printed order form is widely used. It simplifies the ordering procedure.

Ordinarily, orders are not acknowledged unless there is a particular reason for doing so: such, for example, as the need to delay the shipment for some reason; the need to explain why a particular item of the order cannot be shipped; the need to write about terms of payment and shipment; the need to advise the customer that a certain item is not in stock; the need for additional information; the need to refuse an order, etc.

Where an order can be filled without any difficulty, it is regarded as wasteful to acknowledge it. It is, however, advisable to confirm an order in writing that has been placed by telephone or telegram.

The letters that follow are examples of the different kinds of letters that are concerned with placing, acknowledging, confirming, requesting information, accepting or refusing orders.

1580 Valley Road
Peoria, Illinois   61601
March 5, 19___

Globe Department Store
2120 South Shore Drive
Chicago, Illinois 60615

Gentlemen:

Please send me by parcel post six pairs of ladies' nylon hose, size 9½, suntan color, 15 gauge, 65 denier, medium length, reinforced heels and toes.

I am enclosing a check for $9.00, the price you advertised in today's *Tribune*.

Very truly yours,

(Mrs.) Jane Winters

Enc.

(Letter placing an order)

ALBANY SCHOOL FOR ADULTS
3485 MAIN STREET
ALBANY, NEW YORK 12201

August 6, 19___

Monarch Press
Simon & Schuster Building
1230 Avenue of the Americas
New York, New York 10020

Purchase Order No. 43167

Gentlemen:

Please ship by book post and charge to our account the following books listed in your current school catalog:

Quantity		Publication	Unit Price	Amount
25	Cass:	Reading Power Book 1	$2.95	$73.75
20	Cass:	Reading Power Book 2	2.95	59.00
15	Cass:	Reading Power Book 3	3.50	52.50
20	Cass:	Reading Power Book 4	3.50	70.00
				$255.25

We must have these books by September 7, the beginning of the school term.

Very truly yours,

William G. Malone
Principal

(Another letter placing an order)

34

120 East Platte Avenue
Colorado Springs, Colo. 80901
November 10, 19__

Colonial Furniture Company
1050 South Broadway
Denver, Colo. 80202

Gentlemen:

This is to confirm the telephone order I placed this afternoon for the following:

2 walnut bookcases, style number 36-42-18, finished in cordovan, at $85.00 each.

These bookcases are to be delivered in three weeks.

Very truly yours,

Robert Keating

Robert Keating

(Letter confirming a telephone order)

THE YALE MANUFACTURING COMPANY
3120 Railroad Street
New Haven, Conn. 06510

September 8, 19__

Mr. Jerome R. Murphy, Jr.
Trade Associates, Inc.
86 Wintergreen Avenue
Providence, R.I. 02904

Dear Mr. Murphy:

Thank you for your order of September 6, Order No. 43768, for 20 refrigerators, Item No. 381-736. This merchandise is being crated now and will be shipped by tractor-trailer this week. It should arrive at your warehouse before September 15, well in advance of the delivery date you specified.

We have furnished your firm top quality household equipment at reasonable prices for many years. It is our desire to continue to do so.

Please call upon us for any advice or assistance regarding our products. We are anxious to be of service.

Sincerely yours,

Martin T. Harris

Martin T. Harris
Sales Manager

(Letter acknowledging an order)

THE YALE MANUFACTURING COMPANY
3120 Railroad Street
New Haven, Conn. 06510

Dear Customer:

Thank you for your order #............dated........

for...

It will be shipped on.................by..........

We appreciate the opportunity to serve you.

Very truly yours,

Sales Manager

(Card acknowledging an order)

THE HANOVER PICTURE FRAME COMPANY
1432 WOODLAWN ROAD
NASHVILLE, TENNESSEE 37202

April 10, 19__

Miss Marilyn Moss
268 Meadow Lane
Memphis, Tenn. 38101

Dear Miss Moss:

Thank you for your order of April 8 for one dozen picture frames, size 12" by 16", catalog no. 13-126.

These frames come in four different finishes: ebony, walnut, mahogany and maple. Please indicate on enclosed form which finish or finishes you want and return it to us in the enclosed business reply envelope.

Your prompt cooperation will enable us to meet the delivery date you specified.

Sincerely yours,

Oscar Wagner

Oscar Wagner
Manager

Enc.

(Letter requesting additional information about an order)

REGAL TYPEWRITER COMPANY
16847 Ribbon Road ◆ Hartford, Conn. 06101

May 24, 19__

Mrs. Frances R. Hill
682 Revere Avenue
Boston, Mass. 02109

Dear Mrs. Hill:

Thank you for your order of May 20 for one portable Regal Typewriter, Model GK.

The tremendous demand for this typewriter model these past few weeks has depleted our stock. We have wired for additional machines and expect a new supply from our district warehouse within two weeks.

The attractive design, sturdy construction, handsome finish and matching streamlined carrying case have made these machines popular gifts for the high school graduates, as well as for the college students.

Your Regal Typewriter will be delivered to you before June 15. We appreciate your patience in waiting just a little while longer for the model you want.

Cordially yours,

Richard Jackson

Richard Jackson
Sales Manager

(Letter regarding delivery of an order)

35

GENERAL TELEVISION CORPORATION

1914 Circuit Road   ◆   Buffalo, New York 14205

October 7, 19__

Mr. Allen Watts
42-67 Mt. Hope Avenue
Rochester, New York 14603

Dear Mr. Watts:

We appreciate your order of October 4 for our General Television
Set, Model 20 CD. However, our products are distributed only through
authorized dealers.

We are returning your order and check and suggest that you visit
any one of the following General Television dealers in your city.

        ABC Radio and Television Company
        358 Main Street
        Rochester, New York

        Cambridge Television Corporation
        325 Campus Road
        Rochester, New York

        National Appliance Company
        135 Liberty Street
        Rochester, New York

The model you have selected is one of our most popular models on
the market. We know that you will be delighted with this set. The men
who install and service our sets are highly trained technicians who have
completed our intensive training course.

Our dealers will be happy to provide you with the model you have
selected.

                                        Sincerely yours,

                                        William Picker
                                        Sales Manager

Enc.

(Letter refusing an order)

36

CAMBRIDGE TELEVISION CORPORATION
325 CAMPUS ROAD
ROCHESTER, NEW YORK 14604

October 20, 19__

Mr. Allen Watts
42-67 Mt. Hope Avenue
Rochester, New York   14603

Dear Mr. Watts:

Thank you for your order of October 17 for our Cambridge Television
Set, Model 19CQ.

We discontinued this model several months ago. However, our
Model 19CR is an improved model with the added feature of remote
control tuning. It is only $16.50 more than the model you requested.

This added convenience will make television viewing a more enjoyable
experience for the entire family.

We have set aside for you one Cambridge Television Set, Model 19CR
It meets all requirements specified in your original order plus remote
control tuning. We will make immediate delivery as soon as you let us
know on enclosed card that you would like to have this improved model.

Sincerely,

Gerald Watson
Sales Manager

Enc.

(Letter suggesting a substitute for merchandise ordered)

1. Using a mail order catalog or a recent advertisement appearing in your local newspaper, write a letter ordering several household items you need for your home.

2. Assume that you are employed with a large mail order concern. You have just received an order from a new customer for several household items. Write an appropriate letter acknowledging the order.

3. Assume that you are the buyer for a large department store. You have just placed a fairly large order by telephone and are concerned that your order may have been misunderstood. Write a letter confirming the recent order placed by telephone.

4. As an employee of a local department store, you have just received an order for several items of office supplies. You can fill the bulk of the order but have not been given sufficient information regarding the following items:

   Pencils — hardness not indicated in order
   Envelopes — size requirement not shown
   Carbon paper — quantity desired not indicated.

   Write an appropriate letter requesting the additional information.

5. You, an employee of a large bookstore, have received an order for several different books. You can fill the order except for one book which you expect to receive from the publisher in two weeks. Write a letter indicating a delay in delivery of this book.

6. You, an employee in the local department store, have received an order for a set of plated flatware, service for 12, pattern Dawn. You no longer carry the pattern requested although you have a large selection of plated flatware. Prepare an appropriate reply.

7. Assume that you are employed in the mail order department of a company. You have received an order for a product which is not carried by the company. Prepare a letter refusing the order.

8. An order for seasonal merchandise has been received. This merchandise is no longer in stock and no replenishment is expected. Prepare an appropriate reply.

LETTERS REGARDING REMITTANCES

Modern business methods and the widespread use of machines in accounting and shipping have largely diminished the need for letters of transmittal with payments. However, such letters are still used in transactions with local business firms and with individuals who render technical or professional services.

A letter of transmittal should indicate the amount and nature of the enclosure (check or money order or currency) and should give the date of the bill being paid, as well as its number. An expression of appreciation for service rendered is always fitting.

Sometimes payment cannot be made because of an error in a bill or a statement, or because of a misunderstanding as to terms or discounts. Sometimes a check or money order cannot be deposited for payment because it has not been properly signed or there is some other irregularity that prevents the recipient from depositing it. All letters regarding delays in payment should be written promptly but should be tactful, calm and courteous in tone.

As in the case of the letter of transmittal, a letter acknowledging receipt of payment is also not absolutely necessary. However, it may be sent to express appreciation or reassure the payer.

Claims of errors in billing should be investigated carefully and acknowledged as soon as possible. If an error has been made in billing, admit it, apologize and indicate the adjustment to be made, enclosing a corrected bill with the letter of acknowledgment. If no error has been made, explain why the claim is without merit and express appreciation for the opportunity to clear up the misunderstanding.

If it is necessary to ask a bank to stop payment of a check, it should be done promptly, either by telephone or letter. All essential information should be included in a letter requesting that payment of a check be stopped: the check number, date of check, name of payee and amount of check. Where the drawer of the check has a bank account number, this should also be given.

Louise T. Cameron
171-18 135 Avenue
Flushing, New York 11358

April 19, 19__

Dr. George Halleron
853 Holly Avenue
Flushing, N.Y. 11355

Dear Dr. Halleron:

I am enclosing a check for $90.00 for professional services rendered, as shown in your statement dated April 9.

I am grateful for your patience and consideration these past few weeks in connection with the dental work I required.

Gratefully,

Louise F. Cameron

Louise F. Cameron

(Letter enclosing check in payment)

GEORGE HALLERON, D.D.S.
853 Holly Avenue
Flushing, New York 11355

April 22, 19__

Mrs. Louise T. Cameron
171-18 135 Avenue
Flushing, N.Y. 11358

Dear Mrs. Cameron:

Thank you for your check dated April 19 for $90.00.

You were a good patient and I am reasonably sure that you will have no major dental problems for a long time.

Sincerely,

George Halleron

George Halleron, D.D.S.

(Letter acknowledging payment)

GRACE R. CARROLL
115 HOMEWOOD AVENUE
RACINE ● WIS. 53401

July 7, 19__ .

Dr. Robert King
432 Pine Street
Racine, Wis. 53404

Dear Dr. King:

I have just received your statement dated July 4, amounting to $120.00 for professional services rendered during June.

You had told me previously that the fee for the dental work involved would be $100.00. Was an error made in the statement you sent me?

Sincerely,

Grace R. Carroll

Grace R. Carroll

(Letter regarding error in bill or statement)

ROBERT KING, D.D.S.
432 Pine Street
Racine, Wisconsin 53404

July 10, 19__

Mrs. Grace R. Carroll
115 Homewood Avenue
Racine, Wis. 53401

Dear Mrs. Carroll:

I have just received your letter of July 7 and am grateful that you wrote me.

You are correct in stating that I told you my fee would be $100.00. The additional $20.00 was for filling a cavity in your son's tooth on June 3 and for prophylactic treatment of his mouth on June 10.

The statement sent to you should have itemized these additional charges. The total of $120.00, however, is correct.

Sincerely, yours,

Robert King

Robert King, D.D.S.

(Letter explaining seeming discrepancy in amount of bill)

EDUCATIONAL PRESS
711 ACADEMY ROAD
EL PASO, TEXAS 79910

October 15, 19__

Mr. Jack Parker
31 Elm Road
Waco, Texas 76701

Dear Mr. Parker:

We have just received your check for $90.00 in payment of our invoice of October 3. However, we notice that the check was not signed.

We are returning the check for your signature. Please send the signed check back to us in enclosed envelope.

Sincerely,

R. Q. Smith

R.Q. Smith
Chief, Accounting Section

(Letter returning an unsigned check)

---

180 Riverside Drive
New York, N.Y. 10024
August 8, 19__

North River Bank
144 Wall Street
New York, N.Y. 10007

Gentlemen:

Please stop payment on check no. 547, dated August 7, 19__, payable to Metropolitan Lamp Company for $59.79. My bank account number is 4-22170-2.

Very truly yours,

Harold Rowe

Harold Rowe

(Letter stopping payment of a check)

```
Gentlemen:

        Thank you for your check for $321.50 in payment of
our invoice dated March 5.

        We are glad to allow you the 2% cash discount in
this instance.  However, we must remind you that such
discounts are given only when payment is made within
ten days from the date of the invoice.

        We hope that you will be able to take advantage of
our 2% cash discount terms in the future by making pay-
ment during the 10-day period following the invoice date.

                        Very truly yours,
```

(Letter allowing discount deducted)

```
Gentlemen:

        Your check for $321.50 in payment of our invoice
dated March 5 for $328.06 is appreciated.  However, we
cannot allow the 2% discount deducted.

        You realize, of course, that the 2% cash discount
is a premium for prompt payment and can be deducted only
when payment is made within ten days from the date of the
invoice.  We hope you understand why we cannot allow such
discount unless you comply with these terms.

        We are returning your check and request that you send
us a check for the full amount of $328.06.

                        Very truly yours,
```

(Letter disallowing discount deducted)

```
Gentlemen:

        We have received your check for $321.50 in payment
of our invoice dated March 5 for $328.06.  However, we
cannot allow the 2% discount deducted as payment was made
two weeks after the expiration of the ten-day discount
period.

        Under our terms of 2 percent 10 days, net 30, discounts
are allowed only if payment is made within ten days from
the date of the invoice.

        We are crediting the $321.50 to your account.  Will
you please send us an additional check for $6.56 to cover
the balance.

                        Very truly yours,
```

(Another letter disallowing discount deducted)

PRACTICE EXERCISES

1. Assume that you have just been billed for office supplies ordered from a local department store. You know that additional information was needed as your original order was incomplete. You also appreciate the expeditious handling of your order by the department store. Write a letter to accompany your payment by check for $326.85.

2. You are a local storekeeper and have just received payment by check from a new customer. Although delivery of the items he had ordered was delayed for several weeks, the customer made prompt payment. Prepare an appropriate letter acknowledging payment.

3. Assume that you have received Invoice No. 678 of recent date for furniture delivered a week ago by a local furniture dealer. Although the amount for each item is correct, the addition totaled $327.17 instead of $317.17. Prepare a letter to the furniture dealer informing him of the billing error.

4. You, a furniture dealer, have received a letter from one of your customers. He alleges that an error was made in Invoice No. 678 and that the correct amount should be $317.17 instead of $327.17. You ascertain that the customer's claim is justified. Prepare an appropriate reply.

5. You, an employee of a large department store, have received a check from a customer for $321.98 in payment of an invoice sent to him for $336.98. A note accompanying his check stated that he was deducting the shipping charge. You ascertain that the shipping charge should be paid. Prepare an appropriate reply.

LETTERS REGARDING PAST DUE ACCOUNTS

Most business firms and individuals keep their accounts in good order, that is, they pay their bills within the specified terms. However, when credit customers fail to pay their bills long after the terms have expired, it is necessary to send special collection letters.

With regard to credit standing and payment of bills, customers are generally classified as follows:

1. *Good credit risks:* These pay promptly and require little attention. They are given extra time in which to pay before they are sent even a mild reminder of an unpaid bill.
2. *Fair credit risks:* Although these generally pay promptly, they often fall behind in their payments. These too are given extra time in which to pay before a collection reminder is sent.
3. *Poor credit risks:* These have a "marginal" credit rating because they are frequently delinquent in meeting their financial obligations. The accounts of such customers are a cause of concern and they need to be watched. A firm but courteous collection letter is sent as soon as the account becomes overdue.

After the bill, the collection procedure starts with the monthly statement. If, after a fair period of time, payment is not received, further reminders are sent. The frequency and number of these reminders in letter form depend on the amount involved, the length of time the account is overdue and the credit standing of the customer.

Sometimes special notations are rubber-stamped on a statement, reading: PLEASE, or PLEASE REMIT or PAST DUE; at other times, gummed labels with similar word reminders are affixed to the statement. It is when an account becomes seriously past due that the collection letter is used. If the account remains delinquent, it may be necessary to send out a series of collection letters. No matter how stern the letter or how delinquent the account, it must always be written with tact and be courteous in tone. It would be unwise to lose a customer or create ill will while attempting to collect money due.

Following are examples of five collection letters. You will note how the tone becomes more severe with each letter, and yet expresses patience and a desire to cooperate.

THE GREAT WESTERN TRADING CORPORATION
824 WILSHIRE BOULEVARD
LOS ANGELES   ◆   CALIFORNIA 90052

November 15, 19__

Mr. George Spencer
1551 Ocean Avenue
Santa Monica, California 90048

Dear Mr. Spencer:

In looking over our accounts, we find that there is an unpaid balance of $175.00 due us for purchases you made in September. Possibly you have overlooked it.

May we have your check at your earliest convenience? If you have already mailed the check, thank you - and just disregard this letter.

Sincerely yours,

Robert E. Ford

Robert E. Ford
Credit Manager

(First collection letter)

The second letter is a more emphatic reminder. Note that the letter suggests a possible reason why payment has not been made. This is done to appeal to the customer's pride and sense of fairness.

Dear Mr. Spencer:

Although we wrote you on November 15 regarding a balance of $175.00 due for purchases made more than two months ago, we have not yet received your response.

Is there any special reason why payment has not been made? We would appreciate your writing to us or, if you prefer, calling me up. My telephone number is 347-4210.

Let us hear from you soon.

Sincerely,

(Second collection letter)

The last three letters, you will note, are more tersely expressed and the complimentary closings range from *Yours sincerely,* to *Cordially yours,* to *Regretfully yours.* This last letter says that unless payment is received, the account will be turned over to an attorney for collection, as a last resort.

PLEASE — Protect Your Credit ... Honor this Statement

Thank You — WE SINCERELY VALUE YOUR BUSINESS

A Friendly Reminder — THAT YOUR REMITTANCE ON THIS INVOICE IS PAST DUE

Your Payment — WILL BE GREATLY APPRECIATED

HELP! — WE NEED YOUR PAYMENT. WON'T YOU PLEASE MAIL THE FULL AMOUNT TODAY?

Is there a reason — WHY YOU HAVE NOT PAID THIS PAST-DUE AMOUNT? PLEASE CONTACT US IF THERE IS A PROBLEM

A Partial Payment — ON THIS PAST-DUE ACCOUNT WOULD BE APPRECIATED ... IF YOU CANNOT PAY IN FULL TODAY

FINAL NOTICE — Unless you pay this account in full today, we will be forced to place it in the hands of our collection agent.

PAST DUE — YOUR ACCOUNT IS CONSIDERABLY PAST DUE. PLEASE REMIT IMMEDIATELY!

42

Dear Mr. Spencer:

We would like to remind you again that you owe us $175.00 for items purchased in September.

Please give this matter your prompt attention. Your cooperation will be appreciated.

Yours sincerely,

(Third collection letter)

Dear Mr. Spencer:

We regret that we must again remind you of your unpaid balance of $175.00 that has been past due for several months.

We opened a credit account for you and served you to the best of our ability. You agreed to comply with our terms and conditions--namely, to make payment the month following the purchase date. We have been fair with you. Have you been fair with us?

Please send us your check for $175.00 immediately.

Cordially yours,

(Fourth collection letter)

Dear Mr. Spencer:

Although we have, during the past months, sent you many reminders of your overdue account, you have continued to ignore them. You have not even extended to us the courtesy of an acknowledgement or an explanation of your silence.

We now inform you that unless we receive a check for the full amount (175.00) within a week from the date of this letter, we will be forced to turn your account over to our attorneys.

Regretfully yours,

(Fifth collection letter)

If a credit customer replies to a reminder notice or a collection letter that he is unable to make payment at this time and requests a little additional time, write a considerate letter indicating willingness to cooperate. However, state clearly that payment will be expected on the date promised by the customer.

Dear Mr. Spencer:

We have received your letter of January 10 requesting 30 additional days within which to pay the $175.00 due us for purchases you made last September.

We are happy to cooperate and will grant you the extra time you asked for in which to make full payment.

We hope that this extension will be of help to you and look forward to receiving your payment.

Cordially,

REVIEW

1. Name the three classes of credit risks.
2. Which class of credit risk is of most concern to a firm? Why?
3. Name some of the factors that determine the timing of reminder notices.
4. Is obtaining payment of a past due account the only purpose of collection notices and letters? Explain.
5. At which point in the collection letters would you say that the appeal is to fair play and good will?
6. At what point in the collection letters is there a warning?
7. Why should the tone in a series of collection letters become increasingly severe with each letter?
8. Should all delinquent customers be treated alike? Explain.

LETTERS OF COMPLAINT AND ADJUSTMENT

A business receives many different kinds of complaints. It must handle them and "make adjustments" in different ways.

Complaints can be about poor service, damaged, defective or poor quality merchandise, undue delay in receiving orders, mistakes in billing, receiving merchandise other than that ordered, discourteous treatment — and a host of others.

It can be seen that adjusting complaints requires patience, good humor, good manners, the ability to handle difficult problems with ease and promptness — and all of these must come from a sincere desire to be of service to the customer and retain his good will.

In writing letters about complaints and adjustments, there is no room for sarcasm, bitterness, or distrust on the part of the customer. All information as to dates, order numbers, invoice numbers, descriptions of merchandise, methods of shipment, quantities, etc., must be specific and must be carefully checked.

An example of a letter of complaint and two examples of letters of adjustment follow.

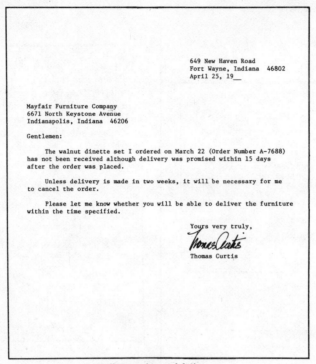

(Letter of complaint)

The message-reply form is particularly useful in following up on orders that have not been delivered. It serves not only as a reminder to the vendor but enables the vendor to explain the reason for the undue delay to the vendee. Both parties will have identical records of the original message and the reply.

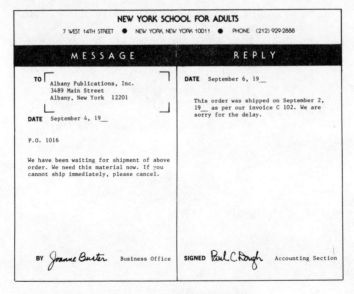

(Message-reply follow-up on order)

44

MAYFAIR FURNITURE COMPANY

6671 NORTH KEYSTONE AVENUE
INDIANAPOLIS, INDIANA 46206

April 27, 19__

Mr. Thomas Curtis
649 New Haven Road
Fort Wayne, Indiana 46802

Dear Mr. Curtis:

Your letter of April 25 reached me this morning. I am sorry to learn that the dinette set you ordered on March 22 has not been delivered and regret the inconvenience it has caused you.

The furniture was shipped from our Gary plant on March 25 and should have been delivered ten days later. The delay was apparently due to transit difficulties.

We have checked with the transit authorities and are assured that the shipment will reach Fort Wayne in two days. We will make every effort to have the dinette set delivered to you on April 30.

Please accept my apologies for the delivery delay and my appreciation for bringing the matter to my attention.

Sincerely yours,

George Kane
Manager

(Letter adjusting a valid complaint)

PAUL JONES CLOTHES, Inc.
1375 Roosevelt Boulevard
Philadelphia ◆ Pennsylvania 19103

May 18, 19__

Mr. Alan Russell
121 Market Street
Camden, New Jersey 08102

Dear Mr. Russell:

We have received the suit and your letter of May 14 requesting a refund of $125.00. You claim the suit does not fit properly.

Our tailor informs me that the suit you returned shows definite sign of wear and, therefore, cannot be put back in stock for resale. Under such circumstances, we cannot make any refund although we would certainly like to please you.

Perhaps some minor alterations will give you the fit you desire. We will be happy to have our tailor alter the suit in accordance with your wishes.

We suggest that you come in and talk it over with Mr. Ted Page, our tailor. He has your suit and has been told to expect you.

We appreciate your bringing this matter to our attention and assure you that our tailor will alter the suit to your satisfaction.

Sincerely yours,

Paul London

Paul London
Manager

(Letter adjusting an invalid complaint)

1. Assume that you recently purchased an electric appliance, such as a toaster, from a department store. You note that it does not operate when you plug it in. You realize that it is an a-c electric appliance although your home is wired for d-c electricity. Prepare an appropriate letter to the department store requesting that some adjustment be made.

2. The bedroom furniture you ordered a month ago from a reputable furniture dealer was delivered yesterday. In checking the various pieces of furniture, you notice that the rear right leg of the night table is cracked. All other pieces appear to be satisfactory. Prepare a letter of complaint.

3. You have just received a letter of complaint from an old customer who recently bought an expensive set of china. She claims that when delivery was made, she found that five cups, four saucers and three soup dishes were cracked. It will take some time to investigate this claim. Prepare a letter of acknowledgment indicating that the matter is receiving careful consideration.

4. Assume that you are in charge of customer relations in a department store. You have received a letter of complaint regarding a file cabinet which was recently delivered to a customer. He alleges that he specified a mahogany finish but received one in a walnut finish. You ascertain that his complaint is justified. Prepare an appropriate reply.

5. You have received a letter of complaint from an irate customer that the 9' x 12' rug she had purchased was faded. She insists that the rug be replaced immediately. You ascertain that the rug was bought more than three years ago, that the rug came from a reputable manufacturer and that no previous complaints had been received regarding this type of rug. Prepare an appropriate reply.

LETTERS REGARDING EMPLOYMENT

Applying for the position

There are two kinds of letters of application for employment that you can write. The first is a letter answering an advertisement. The second is one that you yourself write to a particular firm where you think there may be an opening for you.

In writing a letter of application bear in mind the following: Your letter must *look good*. It must be neatly and accurately typed on good quality paper, with generous margins all around. It must be written in good English, arranged in orderly paragraphs and punctuated intelligently. Remember that your letter of application is really your "work portrait" so be sure to mention everything about your background, your education and your experience. This information will serve to inform the reader about yourself and at the same time give you a better chance of obtaining the job you want.

In certain instances you might want to include what is known as a *personal record sheet* or *résumé*. If you do this then your letter of application can be brief, in the form of a "forwarding letter" for the *résumé*.

Following are two letters of application and a sample personal record sheet or *résumé*.

Several examples of answers to letters of application are also given.

```
                                         312 West 18 Street
                                         New York, N.Y.  10011
                                         October 6, 19__


Columbia Dye Corporation
270 Park Avenue
New York, N.Y.  10017

                        Attention:  Mr. William Meyer

Gentlemen:

     I was very pleased to see your advertisement for an experienced
secretary in today's New York Times.  Here are my qualifications:

     Graduated from Seward Park High School; received secretarial
training at Commercial Business College in New York City.

     Age 28, unmarried, living home with my parents.

     Stenographic speed, 160 words per minute; typing speed, 80 words
per minute.

     Secretary, six years, Universal Match Corporation, where I am
employed at present. This company, now located at 99 Lexington
Avenue, New York, N.Y. 10016, will be moving to Connecticut shortly.
This is why I am seeking other employment.  At present I am secretary
to Mr. Eugene McCoy, Advertising Manager (Telephone:  Longacre 5-6203).

     Stenographer, two years, Dow Toys, Inc., 380 Madison Avenue, New
York, N.Y. 10017.  I worked for Mr. Michael Grant, Credit Manager
(Telephone:  Chelsea 3-5701).

     Please feel free to check with my present employer.  Mr. McCoy
is anxious for me to obtain suitable employment with a reputable firm
before the Universal Match Corporation moves to Connecticut.  I be-
lieve that he will tell you that I have the ability, experience,
personality and appearance necessary for the type of secretary that
is an asset to any organization.

     May I be given the opportunity of an interview?

                                 Sincerely yours,

                                 Dorothy Newman

                                 (Miss) Dorothy Newman
```

(Letter of application answering an advertisement)

```
                                         9 Stuyvesant Oval
                                         New York, N.Y.  10009
                                         January 5, 1979


Personnel Manager
National Foods, Inc.
30 Rockefeller Plaza
New York, N.Y.  10021

Dear Sir:

Your company has been suggested to me as one which might have need for a
person with my technical background.  I believe that my qualifications are
such that I would be particularly useful as a research chemist in your
company.

My resume is attached.  Please note that:

   1.  My graduate specialization was in analytical organic chemistry.

   2.  My undergraduate major was in chemistry with a minor in biology.

   3.  My laboratory experience has been in research, quality control
       and routine food analysis.

If you should have an opening for someone with my qualifications, I would
greatly appreciate a personal interview at your convenience.

                                 Very truly yours,

                                 Donald B. King

                                 Donald B. King

Enc.
```

(Unsolicited letter of application enclosing résumé)

Acknowledging the letter of application

Acknowledgements need not be sent to all applicants for employment. However, applications from persons with desirable qualifications whom you wish to consider for immediate or future employment should be acknowledged with a brief note. If you ask the applicant to come for an interview, be certain to indicate the date, place and time.

```
                                         October 8, 19__


Miss Dorothy Newman
312 West 18 Street
New York, N.Y.  10011

Dear Miss Newman:
```
```
     Your letter applying for the position of Secretary
arrived this morning, and I have read it with considerable
interest.

     Please come for an interview in Room 401 on Thursday,
October 11, between 9 a.m. and 11 a.m.
```

or

```
     Thank you for your letter of October 6.  Although you
appear to have excellent qualifications, they do not meet
our present requirements.

     Should there be an opening in the future for one
with your qualifications, we will get in touch with you.
```
```
                                 Cordially yours,

                                 William Meyer

                                 William Meyer
                                 Business Manager
```

RÉSUMÉ

Donald B. King
9 Stuyvesant Oval
New York, N.Y. 10009

Phone: (212) 673-8338

Vocational Aim:
   To engage in chemical research with a large food manufacturing
organization.

Personal Data:
      Date of Birth: August 1, 1956
      Place of Birth: South Orange, New Jersey
      Marital Status: Single
      Height: 6'1"
      Weight: 175 lbs
      State of Health: Excellent

Education:
      1977 - 1978 New York University, New York, New York.
                   Master of Science degree, September 1978; major, analytical
                   organic chemistry. (Thesis: Microanalytical Techniques
                   for Detecting Food Contaminants)

      1973 - 1977 State University of New York, State University at Buffalo,
                   Buffalo, New York.
                   Bachelor of Science degree, June 1977 (summa cum laude,
                   departmental honors in chemistry). Major in chemistry;
                   minor in biology.

      1970 - 1973 Bronx High School of Science, Bronx, New York.
                   Graduated in June 1973.

Experience:
   October 1978 to date: Chemist with Environmental Protection Project,
Department of Chemistry, New York University, Washington Square, New York,
New York 10003.

   Research work in detection of environmental pollutants with research
project funded by federal grants.

   Summer of 1977: Assistant chemist with General Foods Company, 281
Newark Avenue, Jersey City, New Jersey 07302.

   Engaged in quality control work in connection with the manufacturing of
various food products.

   Summer of 1976: Chemical assistant with Dairy Products, Inc., 306
Lawrence Avenue, Paterson, New Jersey 07510.

   Assisted in routine chemical testing of milk and milk products.

Professional Organizations:
   Member of the American Chemical Society, Association of Food
Technologists and American Association for the Advancement of Science.

Sports and Hobbies:
   Tennis, hiking and photography.

References Furnished on Request

Follow-up by the applicant

If you are particularly interested in a position for which you have applied, you can follow it up with a letter. This letter may be sent after you have submitted your application or after the interview. You may even want to write a follow-up letter where you have been told that there is no vacancy at present, but that your application will be kept on file and will be considered should a vacancy occur.

If you do not receive an acknowledgement of your application within a week or two, you may write a letter of inquiry. Your note should include the following: the date of your application and the position applied for; your interest in the position and your ability to perform the required duties; and a request for information as to the status of your application.

The letter sent after the interview should express your pleasure in meeting the interviewer and your appreciation of the courtesies extended. Include any additional facts you may have omitted in the interview.

Acknowledgement of your application without an immediate offer of employment indicates that your application is being kept on file and may be considered when a vacancy occurs. Your follow-up letter after receiving such an acknowledgement should express appreciation of it, should affirm your interest in becoming associated with the firm, and end with the hope that your application will be given favorable consideration should a vacancy occur.

Checking references

It is customary to check the references of a person who has applied for a position. This usually takes the form of a letter requesting information as to the applicant's abilities, personality, character, fitness for the job, etc.

In answering such a request for information about an applicant, it is of course necessary to be courteous and truthful. Most important, however, such a letter should be considerate, not only of the employer, but of the employee — the person who has applied for the position.

For example, if the applicant was an excellent employee, it is easy to say so in generous terms. If the applicant was a good employee, but had an undesirable trait or two, the reference can still be favorable. It is not necessary to emphasize an applicant's personal shortcomings unless they are of a serious nature that would have an adverse affect on his usefulness to his employer. All correspondence regarding references and recommendations is regarded as confidential.

Following are two letters: one requests information regarding an applicant who has applied for a position; the other answers with a favorable reference and recommendation.

Dear Mr. Meyer:

On August 6, in response to your advertisement that same day in The New York Times, I applied for the position of Secretary.

I do hope that my application is still being considered. I feel that my special training, experience and secretarial skills qualify me for this particular position and that I will be a valuable asset to your organization.

May I hear from you soon.

Sincerely yours,

(Follow-up letter after submitting application)

Dear Mr. Meyer:

It was a pleasure to discuss with you this morning the aims and organization of your company and the duties of the position for which I applied. I am grateful for the time you spent in showing me the layout of the plant.

It is my firm belief that I will be a valuable asset to your company.

I do hope to receive favorable news from you soon.

Sincerely yours,

(Follow-up letter after interview)

Dear Mr. Meyer:

I appreciate the courtesy of your acknowledging my application for the position of Secretary with your firm.

I am very much interested in secretarial employment with your organization and do hope that this will become possible in the near future.

Sincerely yours,

(Follow-up letter after no immediate offer of employment)

COMMERCIAL ASSOCIATES, Inc.
1245 South Avenue
Plainfield   ♦   New Jersey 07001

October 20, 19__

Mr. Edward Davis, Personnel Director
Textile Corporation of America
190 Madison Avenue
New York, New York 10016

Dear Mr. Davis:

Mr. Donald Butler is being considered for the position of Advertising Manager with this company. In his letter of application, he lists your firm as his most recent employer.

We would appreciate your opinion of Mr. Butler's character, personality, ability to handle important advertising accounts and creativity in advertising matters.

Naturally, all information given us will be kept confidential.

Sincerely,

Norman Crandell
President

(Letter checking a reference given by an applicant)

50

TEXTILE CORPORATION OF AMERICA

190 MADISON AVENUE
NEW YORK, NEW YORK 10016

October 24, 19__

Mr. Norman Crandell, President
Commercial Associates, Inc.
1245 South Avenue
Plainfield, New Jersey 07001

Dear Mr. Crandell:

It is with great pleasure that I recommend Mr. Donald Butler for the position of Advertising Manager in your organization.

Mr. Butler has been with us for many years. He started in a clerical capacity and, through successive promotions, became the Assistant Manager in our Advertising Department, the position he has occupied for the last four years.

He is an able, conscientious and hardworking man who is willing to assume added responsibility. A man of integrity and imagination, he tackles his assignments with enthusiasm and does them well.

Opportunities for promotion in this organization are somewhat limited for persons at Mr. Butler's level. Although we would regret losing him, we would be happy to see him advance in the advertising field.

I honestly believe that he would be an asset to your organization.

Sincerely yours,

Edward Davis

Edward Davis
Personnel Director

(Letter recommending an applicant)

51

1. Assume that while reading the *Help Wanted* section of your local newspaper, you notice a *Want Ad* for a position in which you are interested and for which you believe you are qualified. Write a letter applying for this position.
2. Prepare a personal record sheet for yourself, to be used in connection with an application for employment.
3. A neighbor advises you that a position in which you are interested has just become vacant. Write a letter of application to accompany your personal record sheet.
4. Assume that although two weeks have elapsed since you submitted your application for employment, you have heard nothing from the company. Prepare a suitable follow-up letter.
5. Assume that you have just returned from an interview in connection with your application for employment. You realize that there were several pertinent facts which you had not mentioned in your application or at your interview. Prepare a suitable follow-up letter.
6. In connection with your application for employment, you have just received a reply indicating that you were not selected for the existing vacancy but that your application would be kept on file. You are very anxious to obtain employment with this concern. Prepare a suitable follow-up letter.

Miscellaneous Letters on the Social-Personal Aspects of Modern Business

Accepting or declining an invitation to deliver an address

Whether an invitation to deliver an address before a business or professional group is accepted or declined, whether it is written on the personal stationery of the writer or on his business stationery, it should always be gracious and friendly.

The letter accepting the invitation should confirm the time and place for the delivery of the address. It should also contain all other information that relates to the arrangements.

A letter declining an invitation to deliver an address should express sincere regret, should explain why the invitation is declined and should indicate a willingness to deliver an address at a future date.

It will be my pleasure to address the membership of the Commerce Club at its monthly luncheon meeting on Tuesday, September 18 at 12:30 p.m. at the Malverne Hotel.

The topic, "Automation in Industry," is a broad one and I shall attempt to cover those aspects pertaining to executive management.

The enclosed biographical sketch will provide the information you requested regarding my background.

It is with regret that I must decline your invitation to address the membership of the Commerce Club at its September luncheon meeting.

I have a previous engagement in Rochester on that day and cannot cancel it at this time.

It will be my pleasure to address your group at a subsequent meeting.

Acknowledging a letter that is being referred to someone else for reply

It will sometimes happen that a letter addressed to someone in a business firm needs to be answered by someone else who is particularly familiar with the subject-matter. In such a case, a short, courteous letter of acknowledgement like the following is necessary. Note the specific and specialized nature of the information requested.

UNIVERSAL PAINT COMPANY
123 Enamel Road
Pittsburgh, Pennsylvania   15214

July 29, 19__

Mr. Richard Parker
42 Railroad Avenue
Reading, Pa.   19602

Dear Mr. Parker:

Your letter of July 27 requesting information about acid and alkali-resistant paint has been referred to Dr. Martin Sharp, our Technical Director.

I am certain that you will hear from him shortly.

Sincerely yours,

Joseph Warner

Joseph Warner
Sales Manager

Cancelling an appointment

A letter cancelling an appointment should be written as soon as the situation which makes the cancellation necessary arises. As a matter of courtesy, it is desirable to give the reason for cancelling, and also, when possible, to suggest another time for an appointment.

DIAMOND RUBBER COMPANY

3316 GLEN AVENUE

BALTIMORE   ◆   MARYLAND 21215

December 5, 19__

Mr. Charles Young
2306 May Boulevard
Alexandria, Virginia   22310

Dear Mr. Young:

   Mr. Martin Adams was called away on a special business trip.
He asked me to write that he will be unable to see you on Thursday
but could see you the following Monday during the early afternoon.

   Please let me know if that would be convenient for you.

Sincerely yours,

Pearl Wright

Pearl Wright
for
Mr. Martin Adams

Changing the address for a subscription

When a subscriber to a newspaper or periodical changes his mailing address, he should immediately so notify the publication. This will insure its uninterrupted delivery.

Sometimes, for the convenience of the subscriber, a publication will provide its own printed form to be used in reporting a change of address. Where such a printed form is not provided, a short, direct letter is necessary.

Here are two examples of such change-of-address letters. Note that the second letter attaches a mailing label showing the new address.

Gentlemen:

    I am a subscriber to <u>Sophisticated News</u>. Please note the following change of address, effective May 1:

Old Address: Rose Ann Mallard
                  8 Peter Cooper Road
                  New York, N.Y. 10010

New Address: Rose Ann Mallard
                  85 East End Avenue
                  New York, N.Y. 10028

                  Very truly yours,

---

                  8 Peter Cooper Road
                  New York, N.Y. 10010
                  March 10, 19__

Subscription Department
Sophisticated News
21 Princeton Circle
Camden, N.J. 08101

Gentlemen:

    I am a subscriber of <u>Sophisticated News</u> and wish to inform you that, effective May 1, my new address will be:

        Rose Ann Mallard
        85 East End Avenue
        New York, N.Y. 10028

    I have attached to the bottom of this letter the mailing label for the March issue of <u>Sophisticated News</u>.

            Very truly yours,

            Rose Ann Mallard

            Rose Ann Mallard

```
ROSE ANN MALLARD
8 PETER COOPER RD
NEW YORK NY 10010

WEN 5230 ITH  CS51 2200
```

Confirming a hotel reservation

A letter that confirms a hotel reservation must state clearly the type of accommodation, the rate per day and the period of time. Such a confirming letter should also include any special instructions that may be necessary as to delay in arrival, and end with an expression of good will.

NATIONAL HOTEL
1946 N Street, N.W.
Washington, D.C. 20012

Telephone:
202-344-4444

                May 16, 19__

Mr. Warren Anderson
102 Kalamazoo Street
Lansing, Mich. 48921

Dear Mr. Anderson:

    We have reserved a single room with private bath for you for five days beginning June 24.

    The room with bath is $28.00 a day. Your reservation will be held until 7:00 p.m. on June 24. Should you be delayed, please wire or telephone the approximate arrival time to assure that your reservation is held.

    We look forward to welcoming you at the National Hotel. Our facilities are at your disposal to help make your visit a comfortable and enjoyable one.

        Sincerely,

        William Reed

        William Reed
        Reservation Manager

Congratulating a friend on his promotion

One way to show a friend how you feel when he has been honored with a promotion is to write him a personal letter of congratulation. In such a letter, you have an opportunity to express yourself warmly and to wish him continued success.

    I was delighted to read in today's <u>Times</u> the announcement of your promotion to vice-president of the International Advertising Corporation.

    You certainly deserve this promotion and I congratulate you. Your company is to be commended for its wisdom in selecting you for this important post.

    My best wishes to you and International Advertising for continued success.

Explaining a delay in answering a letter

When a letter addressed to a particular person cannot be answered promptly because of that person's absence, it is good practice for someone, usually the secretary, to send a letter of acknowledgement. Such a letter can explain why the person addressed has been unable to answer, and can offer the assurance that on his return, the letter will be answered fully and without further delay.

June 10, 19___

Mr. Victor Brady
246 Sterling Avenue
New Rochelle, N.Y.   10801

Dear Mr. Brady:

We have received your letter of June 7 addressed to Mr. Robert Jordan.

Mr. Jordan is out of town and is not expected back before June 18.

Please be assured that your letter will be brought to his attention when he returns to the office.

Sincerely,

Hazel Brown

Hazel Brown
Secretary to
Mr. Robert Jordan

Extending holiday greetings

Holiday greetings from business firms, particularly at the Christmas and New Year season, have become a standard custom.

These holiday greetings can take the form of a letter, a special card with the firm's name imprinted, or a personal message from an executive of the firm. Sometimes such a greeting is accompanied by a small gift such as a calendar, a desk appointment book, a novelty pencil, or a paperweight. Such holiday greetings express the spirit of the season and serve to strengthen good will.

The letter that follows on the next page is a straightforward example of a Christmas and New Year letter from the president of a business firm.   Notice the personal note at the end.

Most business firms today send their holiday greetings by means of "greeting cards" rather than letters. There are an infinite variety of them covering all sorts of occasions and holidays.

The custom of sending greeting cards dates back to Biblical times, ancient Rome and even to China, many centuries ago.

It is estimated that today more than six billion greeting cards are mailed annually in the United States. When we realize that this means 110 greeting cards used by each family in a year, it is easy to appreciate their popularity.

In addition to Christmas, the New Year and Easter, greeting cards are sent to express sentiments and good wishes for many holidays, special occasions and personal remembrances. There are greeting cards for national holidays, saints' days, weddings, births, birthdays, best wishes, thank you, health and many others. The cards come in all sorts of sizes, shapes and colors. Some are serious, some are humorous and some are thought-provoking. All are attractively designed and illustrated in ways that are appropriate to the sentiments expressed in them. Many greeting cards are quite beautiful and show genuine artistry. Some people who regard the greeting card as too impersonal, prefer to write their own messages in the form of letters and notes. Even they, however, find the greeting card very handy for sending greetings and wishes on certain occasions.

Following is a list of holidays and special days on which greeting cards are sent.

April Fool's Day, April 1
Pranksters feel that it is permissible to play all sorts of tricks on this day.

Ash Wednesday
The first day of Lent, generally in February or March.

Christmas Day, December 25
This is both a legal and religious holiday. It observes the anniversary of the birth of Jesus. All states and all those of the Christian faith celebrate this holiday.

Columbus Day
The second Monday in October, to commemorate the discovery of America by Columbus in 1492. Prior to 1971, it was celebrated on October 12, the anniversary of the discovery.

Easter
The first Sunday after the first full moon that occurs at the end of the vernal equinox.

Election Day
The first Tuesday after the first Monday in November for the election of public officials. This holiday is observed in most states.

Father's Day
The third Sunday in June, set aside to honor fathers.

Flag Day, June 14
Legal holiday observed in some states. Commemorates the adoption of the flag (Stars and Stripes) by the Continental Congress, in 1777.

Good Friday
The Friday before Easter.

Hallowe'en, October 31
A special day for making merry, wearing costumes and playing old-fashioned games. A favorite with children.

Independence Day, July 4
Legal holiday observed in all states. The Declaration of Independence was adopted on this day, in 1776.

Labor Day
The first Monday in September. Set aside to honor labor, it is a legal holiday in all states.

EMPIRE TRANSPORT COMPANY
884 Empire Boulevard
Jersey City, N. J. 07302

December 18, 19__

Mr. George W. Brady
Community Appliances, Inc.
400 Lincoln Park
Newark, N.J. 07104

Dear Mr. Brady:

The Season's Greetings!

The accompanying desk appointment book is but a small token of our appreciation of your always-welcome patronage. Please accept our assurance that we will continue to give you our best possible service in the months ahead.

Our very best wishes to your family and office staff - to which I add my own greetings to you personally.

Sincerely yours,

Lawrence Allen

Lawrence Allen
President

Lincoln's Birthday, February 12
Legal holiday in many states.

Memorial Day
The last Monday in May, to honor the memory of the dead of all wars. Prior to 1971, it was celebrated on May 30.

Mother's Day
The second Sunday in May, set aside to honor mothers.

New Year's Day, January 1
Legal holiday observed in all states.

Palm Sunday
The Sunday before Easter.

St. Patrick's Day, March 17
Observance of the death of Ireland's patron saint.

Thanksgiving Day
Generally the fourth Thursday in November, set aside for national thanksgiving, especially of our democratic form of government. It is a legal holiday in all states.

Valentine's Day, February 14
Candy, flowers and other tokens of affection are exchanged on this day, in honor of St. Valentine.

Veterans' Day, November 11
Set aside to honor the veterans of the U.S. Armed Forces, it is a legal holiday in all states.

Washington's Birthday
The third Monday in February, in honor of the founder and first President of the United States. Prior to 1971, it was celebrated on February 22.

Special kinds of greeting cards are sent on many of the above holidays. In addition, cards are also sent in recognition and celebration of special occasions and events, as follows:

Anniversary congratulations

Birth announcements

Birth congratulations

Birthday greetings

Engagement congratulations

Friendship cards

Get-well cards

Gift cards

Graduation congratulations

Party invitations

Promotion congratulations

Religious cards (confirmation and ordination)

Retirement congratulations

Success in a new venture

Sympathy and condolence cards

Thank you cards

Trip and travel cards
   (bon voyage)

Wedding congratulations
— and many, many others.

Introducing a person by letter

It is sometimes necessary, in business, to write a personal letter of introduction. This happens when a person is seeking employment in another city or wishes to apply for employment in a particular firm. In both instances, the letter of introduction is written by someone who knows the person to whom the letter is addressed and the person whom it concerns.

Following on the next page is an example of such a letter of introduction. Note that it is brief and to the point.

Making a hotel reservation

Hotel reservations can be made by telephone, by telegram, in person or by letter. The reservation should be placed well in advance to make certain that an accommodation will be available. In writing a letter reserving a hotel room, it is well to give all particulars; that is, to state the length of the stay, the person (or persons) for whom the reservation is being made, the type of accommodation, the time and date of arrival, and the rate per day. It is desirable to request confirmation of the reservation being made.

```
                                    102 Kalamazoo Street
                                    Lansing Mich.  48921
                                    May 12, 19__

National Hotel
1946 N Street, N.W.
Washington, D.C.  20012

Gentlemen:

     Please reserve a single room with private bath for me for five
days starting June 24 at a daily rate of no more than $28.00.

     I should arrive during the late afternoon on June 24.  Please con-
firm this reservation.

                                    Very truly yours,

                                    Warren Anderson
                                    Warren Anderson
```

310 Victory Parkway
Cincinnati, Ohio 45231
October 17, 19__

Mr. Frank Jackson
Commercial Products Corporation
6005 Foster Avenue
Chicago, Illinois 60672

Dear Mr. Jackson:

   This letter is presented by Margaret Ronan who is the daughter of a
close friend of mine.

   She has just moved to Chicago and is looking for a position as a
secretary. She is a young woman of excellent education and background and
is highly qualified to perform the duties of secretary.

   Knowing the nature of your organization, I thought that you might
be able to use the kind of services Miss Ronan has to offer. Anything you
can do for her would be very much appreciated.

                          Gratefully yours,

                          Henry Avery
                          Henry Avery

(Introducing a person by letter)

59

Ordering theater tickets

In a letter ordering theater tickets, it is necessary to give the following information: the title of the play, concert, dance recital, etc.; the date for which the tickets are desired; an alternate date should the first choice be unavailable; whether the tickets are for a matinee or evening performance; the location of the seats; and the price. The letter ordering tickets should be accompanied by check or money order and should include a stamped, self-addressed envelope.

Following is an example of a letter ordering theater tickets.

```
                                      172 Holland Road
                                      South Orange, N.J.  07079
                                      May 10, 19__

Imperial Theater
301 West 44 Street
New York, N.Y.  10036

Gentlemen:

     Please send me four orchestra tickets, at $15.00 each, for the
evening performance of Hamlet on June 5th.  Alternate choices are:  June
12th or June 19th.

     My check for $60.00 and a self-addressed stamped envelope are enclosed.

                                      Very truly yours,

                                      Bernard Horn
                                      Bernard Horn
Encl.
```

Submitting a letter of resignation

If a person wants to resign from an organization, it is often necessary for him to do so by means of a letter. Such a letter serves to make the resignation "official" and also offers an opportunity to explain the reason for resigning. Usually, a letter of resignation is merely a confirmation of a previous mutual understanding between those concerned. Such a letter of resignation should express appreciation of the association that is being terminated and regret at the necessity for doing so.

```
                                      308 Compo Road
                                      Waterbury, Conn.  06702
                                      September 15, 19__

Board of Directors
Johnson Electrical Corporation
1285 Boston Avenue
Bridgeport, Conn.  06603

Gentlemen:

     It is with sincere reluctance that I submit my resignation of the
position I have held the past six years, to take effect on October 30,
19__ .

     My association with the Johnson Electrical Corporation has been a
most pleasant one.  I cannot too warmly express my gratitude for the
consideration I received during my tenure with the company as well as
the personal friendships that I have enjoyed with my associates.

     As I explained at a recent conference, I have received a very at-
tractive offer from another company which I have decided to accept.  The
sizable increase in salary and the opportunities offered for promotion are
my reasons for resigning and making this change.

     May I express my best wishes for the continued success of the com-
pany and the well-being of its staff.

                                      Yours very truly,

                                      James Scott
                                      James Scott
```

Mailgrams, Telegrams, and Other Telegraphic Services

Mailgram messages and telegrams provide the speed, economy and sense of urgency so vital to much of today's business communications. They are used in business and for the transmission of personal messages whenever it is necessary to send a brief, urgent message which is sufficiently important to require documentation and which cannot be accomplished as well by means of a conventional letter.

Telegraphic service can also be used to transmit money and to order such gifts as candy or flowers for special occasions.

Both domestic and international telegraphic services are available.

DOMESTIC TELEGRAPH SERVICE

Telegraphic messages can be filed in person at any Western Union public office or agency. Such messages can also be telephoned from home or office to Western Union and charged to your telephone bill. They may also be sent from a public telephone, at which payment can be made through the coin-slot, on advice as to the amount from the telephone operator. If facsimile or teleprinter machine facilities are available at your office, such messages may be transmitted by Desk-Fax or teletypewriter exchange service (TWX or Telex).

Domestic service is used to transmit messages between any two points in the United States, and between points in the United States and Canada or Mexico. There are two types of domestic telegraph service. These are: (1) Mailgram messages and (2) telegrams.

Mailgram messages

Mailgram service is a joint offering of Western Union and the United States Postal Service. Mailgram messages are physically delivered by letter carriers anywhere in the United States or Canada. There is no extra charge for such service. They are transmitted electronically over Western Union's communications network directly to a U.S. Post Office near the recipient's address. There, the message is typed by high-speed equipment and inserted into a distinctive blue and white envelope for delivery with the next business day's mail.

The general public can relay Mailgram messages to Western Union by telephone or by filing in person at a Western Union public office or agency. Such telephone calls are toll-free and may be made 24 hours a day, seven days a week.

If your office has Telex or TWX, you can readily send Mailgram messages via teletypewriter. The high-volume user, one with a need for fast delivery of large numbers of messages, can have thousands of messages transmitted simultaneously by putting Mailgram messages on magnetic tape. Computer-originated messages may be sent as a common text to many addresses, as a different text to each address or as a common text with variable inserts. Stored Mailgram service provides computer storage of frequently used letter texts, key paragraphs, mailing lists and sender names and titles.

Other services available to high-volume Mailgram users are:

Business reply Mailgram messages. When a written response to your Mailgram message is desired, you can add a reply form at the bottom of your message. The recipient need only fill it in and fold it into an accompanying business reply envelope for mailing back to you.

Certified Mailgram service. When you need to be sure that your message was received, this service will provide a signed receipt returned to you by the U.S. Postal Service.

Telegrams

The full rate telegram is the fastest type of public service message. Two basic types of delivery are provided—messenger and telephone. Messenger delivery, available in most places, is guaranteed within five hours. Phone delivery is guaranteed within two hours, and a written copy of the message can be sent by mail to the recipient. A minimum charge is made for fifteen words or less, with an additional charge for all words beyond that number. There is no charge for the date line including the city and state, the name and address of the recipient or the name of the sender.

The telegram is available for sending and phone delivery 24 hours a day, including Sundays and holidays. Messenger delivery of telegrams is not available everywhere or at all times. Be sure to ascertain availability of messenger delivery when calling Western Union with a telegram to be delivered by messenger. If for any reason a message cannot be delivered, the Western Union office at the destination will

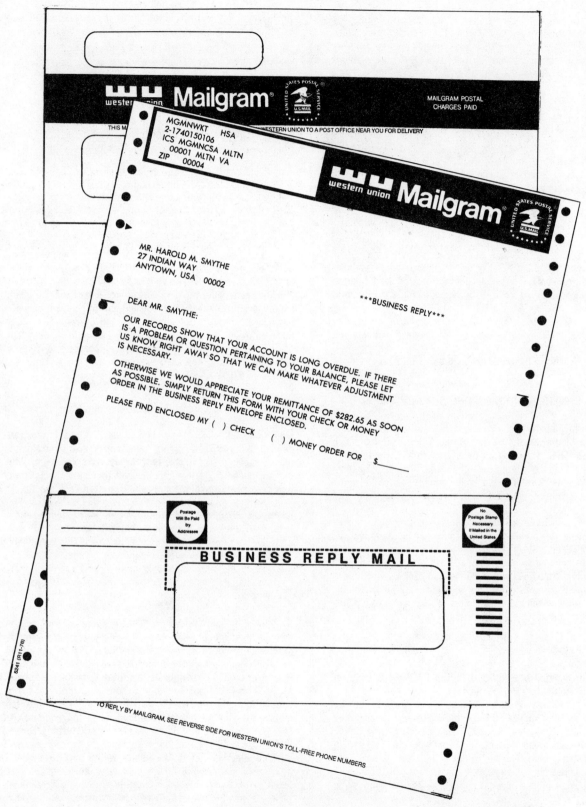

Mailgram ®

western union

MAILGRAM POSTAL
CHARGES PAID

THIS M... ...WESTERN UNION TO A POST OFFICE NEAR YOU FOR DELIVERY

MGMNWKT   HSA
2-1740150106
ICS MGMNCSA MLTN
00001 MLTN VA
ZIP   00004

Mailgram ®

western union

MR. HAROLD M. SMYTHE
27 INDIAN WAY
ANYTOWN, USA 00002

BUSINESS REPLY

DEAR MR. SMYTHE:

OUR RECORDS SHOW THAT YOUR ACCOUNT IS LONG OVERDUE. IF THERE
IS A PROBLEM OR QUESTION PERTAINING TO YOUR BALANCE, PLEASE LET
US KNOW RIGHT AWAY SO THAT WE CAN MAKE WHATEVER ADJUSTMENT
IS NECESSARY.

OTHERWISE WE WOULD APPRECIATE YOUR REMITTANCE OF $282.65 AS SOON
AS POSSIBLE. SIMPLY RETURN THIS FORM WITH YOUR CHECK OR MONEY
ORDER IN THE BUSINESS REPLY ENVELOPE ENCLOSED.

PLEASE FIND ENCLOSED MY ( ) CHECK

( ) MONEY ORDER FOR $_____

Postage
Will Be Paid
by
Addressee

No
Postage Stamp
Necessary
If Mailed in the
United States

BUSINESS REPLY MAIL

5241 (R11-76)

TO REPLY BY MAILGRAM, SEE REVERSE SIDE FOR WESTERN UNION'S TOLL-FREE PHONE NUMBERS

Business reply mailgram service

62

notify the sending office which in turn will notify you.

Other special telegram services are available at varying costs. These are:

Overnight telegram. This service offers message delivery by 2 p.m. the following day. It is priced much lower than the full rate telegram. A minimum charge is made for one hundred words or less, with an additional charge for all words beyond that number.

Repeat-back and valued-message services. These two special services offer financial protection in situations where the telegram has a monetary value in excess of $500.

Repeat-back service is available if the value is $5000 or less. At an additional charge, the receiving office sends the message back to the sending office for verification.

Valued message service is available if the declared value exceeds $5000. A repeat-back is used again, and the sender pays an extra cost of 1/10 of one percent of the declared value.

Personal delivery only service. This special service is provided at no charge to the sender who wants the telegram handed directly to the addressee—and to no one else.

Alternate delivery. If there is a possibility that the telegram may be undelivered at one location, an alternate address may be specified. There is an extra charge for this service.

Confirmation copy. If a written record of the telegram is wanted by the sender, a copy can be furnished as a Mailgram message for a nominal charge.

Report delivery. If the sender wishes confirmation that a telegram has been delivered, whether by telephone or by messenger, a telegram or Mailgram is sent to the originator advising when the message was delivered. The cost for this service is the minimum prevailing rate for a full rate telegram or a base rate Mailgram.

Format for domestic telegraph blanks

Blank telegraph forms are provided free by Western Union. These forms provide space for indicating the following:

1. Type of service desired
2. Payment arrangements
3. Date of origin
4. Name and address of recipient
5. Special instructions
6. Text of message
7. Signature (sender's name)
8. Sender's name, address and telephone number

In filling out the telegraph form, it is preferable to type or print. If the message is handwritten, be certain that the writing is clear and legible.

Preparing the telegraph form for transmission

The essential steps in preparing the sending blank for transmission are as follows:

1. Check the box in the upper right-hand corner if you wish to send an overnight telegram. If box is not checked, the message is sent as a full rate telegram.

2. Place the date at the upper-right side of the blank.

3. Place in the space provided at the upper-left side

the word **PAID** if the sender is paying and **COLLECT** if the recipient of the telegram is to pay.

4. If the sender is not paying cash, indicate the corporation, firm or individual to be charged and the account number in the space provided for such purposes.

5. The name and address of the corporation, firm or individual to whom the telegraphic message is to be sent is placed in the spaces provided at the upper-left side. Be sure to place tieline designation or PHONE after the recipient's name if physical delivery by Western Union messenger is not desired.

6. If any special handling is being requested, it too must be shown immediately following the recipient's name.

7. Start the message below the upper heavy horizontal line and flush with the left-hand margin. The message should be stated clearly and concisely. Avoid ambiguous phrases. Such words as "the," "that," "and," "I," and "a" can generally be eliminated without any loss of meaning. Do not use salutations and complimentary closings such as "Dear Sir" and "Yours truly." There is no charge for punctuation marks in the text of the message.

8. The name of the sender is placed several lines below the message, on the right-hand side of the blank. The name of the firm may be included in the signature.

9. Place the sender's name, address and telephone number below the lower heavy horizontal line in the spaces provided. This information is for reference purposes only.

Telegraphic money orders

Domestic money order service is available for transmitting money to any place within the United States. Two classes of service are available. Day money orders, the more expensive class, are accepted for immediate transmission and delivery. Overnight money orders provide more economical overnight service and are accepted up until midnight for notification of payment to the payee as early as possible the following morning. A message may be included with the money order.

A special form for sending telegraphic money orders is provided by Western Union. In addition to specifying the amount to be paid and the name and address of the person who is to receive the money, the sender may indicate whether a report of payment is wanted and whether or not identification is to be waived when the recipient calls for the money.

Anyone holding a Master Charge or Visa (BankAmericard) credit card may send up to $300 via Western Union anywhere in the forty-eight states. Do not visit any Western Union public office or agency for such service. It must be done by telephone—home, office or public telephone. Such telephone calls are toll-free and may be made 24 hours a day, seven days a week. If sent during business hours of the paying office, the money may be picked up by the recipient within two hours after the telephone order was placed. Supplementary messages cannot be included with charge card money orders.

Telegram

western union · Telegram

MSG. NO.	NO. OF SVC. CL. OF WDS.	PD.-COLL.	CASH NO.	ACCOUNTING INFORMATION	DATE	FILING TIME	SENT TIME
				Diamond Chemical Co. 46938	June 5, 19__	A.M. P.M.	A.M. P.M.

Send the following message, subject to the terms on back hereof, which are hereby agreed to

☐ OVER NIGHT TELEGRAM
UNLESS BOX ABOVE IS CHECKED THIS MESSAGE WILL BE SENT AS A TELEGRAM

TO Walter Parker, Analytical Appliances, Inc.

ADDRESS & TELEPHONE NO. 31 Exchange Street

CITY – STATE & ZIP CODE Rochester, New York

Thank you for your order 817. Analytical equipment and spare parts were shipped this date from our Peoria plant by American Transport Line. Other material will be sent by air mail tomorrow. Please let us know if we can be of additional help.

Raymond C. Bunsen, Diamond Chemical Company

SENDER'S TEL. NO. (312) 673-6202 (Area Code) NAME & ADDRESS Raymond C. Bunsen, Diamond Chemical Company, 32 Hot Plate Circle, Chicago, Illinois 60606

W.U. 5210 (3/73)

Telegram

western union · Telegram

MSG. NO.	NO. OF SVC. CL. OF WDS.	PD.-COLL.	CASH NO.	ACCOUNTING INFORMATION	DATE	FILING TIME	SENT TIME
		Collect			April 1, 19—	A.M. P.M.	A.M. P.M.

Send the following message, subject to the terms on back hereof, which are hereby agreed to

☐ OVER NIGHT TELEGRAM
UNLESS BOX ABOVE IS CHECKED THIS MESSAGE WILL BE SENT AS A TELEGRAM

TO *James Miller (Personal Delivery Only)*

ADDRESS & TELEPHONE NO. *270 Park Avenue*

CITY – STATE & ZIP CODE *New York, New York*

Running out of funds. Wire $250.00 immediately. Staying at Paradise Hotel in Las Vegas. Love.

Thomas Miller

SENDER'S TEL. NO. *(702) 735-4101* (Area Code) NAME & ADDRESS *Thomas Miller, Paradise Hotel, Las Vegas, Nevada* (Zip Code) *89109*

W.U. 5210 (3/73)

SEE IMPORTANT INFORMATION ON THE REVERSE SIDE OF THIS FORM.   PRESS FIRMLY - PRINT CLEARLY.

Telegraphic Money Order

western union

SENDING DATA	CLASS TYPE	OFFICE	WORD COUNT	DATE AND FILING TIME	CLERKS INIT. AND ACCTG. INFORMATION	$	AMT.
							FEE
						S	TOLLS
							RP MGM
MOD		86 078 77=				E	TAX
							TOTAL

DO NOT WRITE ABOVE THIS LINE

PAY AMOUNT: Two Hundred Fifty and   00/100 DOLLARS (250.00) CAU
FIGURES   CAU OR VIG

TO: Thomas Miller   REPORT PAYMENT BY MAILGRAM   YES ☒ NO ☐
(ADDITIONAL CHARGE)

TEST QUESTION: TELEPHONE NO.
STREET ADDRESS AND APT. NUMBER: Paradise Hotel   CITY Las Vegas   STATE: Nev.   ZIP: 89109

SENDER'S NAME: James Miller
SENDER'S STREET ADDRESS AND APT. NO.: 270 Park Avenue   CITY New York   STATE: N.Y.   ZIP: 10017
(IF REPORT PAYMENT REQUESTED)

MESSAGE: Hurry home. All is forgiven.   = MOD =

SENDER'S FULL NAME: James Miller   270 Park Ave. N.Y.N.Y. 10017 (212) 684-6021
ADDRESS   TELEPHONE NO.

WU 72 (R3-77)

● Unless signed below the Telegraph Company is directed to pay this money order at my risk to such person as its paying agent believes to be the above named payee, personal identification being waived. Foreign money orders excepted.

James Miller

⑈086078771⑈ 66

65

If report of payment is requested by the sender, Western Union will advise when the recipient received payment by means of a Mailgram. The Mailgram message will appear as shown below:

YOUR

MONEY ORDER

OF APRIL 2

TO THOMAS MILLER

WAS PAID APRIL 2

Teletypewriters

The teletypewriter is a device that transmits and receives written messages. It is a combination of two communication methods: the telephone and the letter. It is one of the fastest and most efficient means of communication when the need is immediate and a written record is required. Many large companies have their own internal teletypewriter systems, thus permitting instant written communication with their own branch offices. These companies generally have Telex and/or TWX as well.

Modern technology not only enables Telex and TWX subscribers to communicate with each other, it also enables them to:

1. Send multiple address messages, including Mailgram messages by teletypewriter.

2. Use stored texts and address lists

Some important features of Telex and TWX communications are:

1. Teletype communication can take place 24 hours a day, seven days a week. Messages can be received when terminals are unattended, such as during non-office hours.

2. Both sender and receiver get an exact and permanent copy of every message.

3. After dialing Telex-to-Telex, TWX-to-TWX, Telex-to-TWX or TWX-to-Telex, sender can get an automatic identification ("answerback") assuring that desired party has been reached. The automatic identification may be repeated at the end of the transmission confirming that the message was received.

Facsimile

A facsimile transceiver is a device that both transmits and receives a reproduction of a page. Facsimile or "fax" is useful for rapid transmission of materials such as typewritten copy, engineering drawings, charts, maps, photographs, etc. As facsimile-produced materials do not reproduce clearly on office copying equipment, facsimile is used when only one copy is required by the receiver.

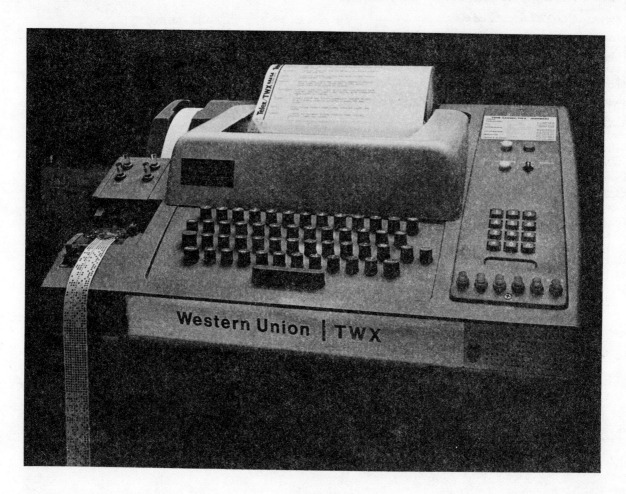

Business correspondence by telegraph

Although written communication in business is mostly by letters, there are times when urgent matters requiring immediate action can be handled with greater ease by telegraphic means. Following are some sample telegraphic messages that may be used in place of business letters.

Inquiring about prices, delivery, availability, etc.:

WIRE PRICE AND BEST SHIPPING DATE FOR THIRTY PORTABLE RECORDERS MODEL K-1217.

WIRE COLLECT IF IMMEDIATE SHIPMENT OF ONE HUNDRED TONS OF TROPICAL BLEACH CAN BE MADE AT REGULAR LIST PRICE.

Placing the order:

SHIP US THE FOLLOWING TO ARRIVE ON OR ABOUT 8/15: ITEM NO. 64821, SIZE 3/4", QUANTITY 1500 FEET ITEM NO. 64825, SIZE 1-1/2", QUANTITY 3000 FEET

Acknowledging the order:

THANK YOU FOR YOUR ORDER 937. MERCHANDISE SHIPPED BY AIREX THIS DATE.

Requesting that delivery be expedited:

OUR ORDER GK-224 URGENTLY NEEDED. PLEASE WIRE EARLIEST POSSIBLE SHIPPING DATE.

Replying to inquiries regarding delivery:

EXPEDITING DELIVERY OF ORDER GK-224. SHIPMENT WILL BE MADE TUESDAY.

RETEL ORDER MD 852 WILL BE SHIPPED 4/16 VIA AIR MAIL SPECIAL DELIVERY.

Encouraging salesmen:

CONGRATULATIONS ON MEETING YOUR MONTHLY SALES QUOTA. KEEP UP THE GOOD WORK.

Promoting sales:

I WISH TO EXPRESS MY PERSONAL APPRECIATION OF YOUR RECENT ORDER GIVEN TO MR. HAROLD FIELDS. SHIPMENT WILL BE MADE FROM OUR REGIONAL WAREHOUSE IN A FEW DAYS. PLEASE LET US KNOW IF WE CAN BE OF ANY ADDITIONAL SERVICE TO YOU. ON YOUR NEXT VISIT TO OUR CITY I WILL BE GLAD TO MEET YOU PERSONALLY.

Collecting overdue accounts:

VERY IMPORTANT THAT YOU WIRE YOUR INTENTIONS RE OUR LETTER NOVEMBER 3.

REMITTANCE OF $695.75 FOR OUR INVOICE OF APRIL 15 WILL BE APPRECIATED. WIRE REPLY.

URGENT WE RECEIVE PAYMENT THIS WEEK. WE VALUE YOUR FRIENDSHIP TOO MUCH TO BE COMPELLED TO RESORT TO LEGAL ACTION.

IMPERATIVE REMITTANCE ON YOUR ACCOUNT BE SENT IMMEDIATELY TO AVOID ACTION BY OUR LAWYERS.

Special social and other domestic telegraph services

For those occasions when you wish to send greetings, congratulations, condolences, invitations or announcements, the domestic telegram is fast and convenient. If time permits, such messages may be sent more economically by Mailgram service. Suggested wordings for such special messages are obtainable from the Western Union Telegraph Company.

Some of the services that the telegraph company offers are:

1. *Candygrams.* It will deliver a box of candy with a telegraph message.
2. *Flowers.* It will wire instructions to the distant city where your order will be promptly delivered by a qualified florist. A card containing a personal message from a sender will be delivered with the flowers.

Following are some suggested messages that may be helpful to you for developing your own messages for those special occasions.

Anniversary:

CONGRATULATIONS ON YOUR ANNIVERSARY. MAY EACH ONE BRING ADDED HAPPINESS.

CONGRATULATIONS AND BEST WISHES FOR LONG LIFE, PROSPERITY, HEALTH AND HAPPINESS.

Bar Mitzvah:

CONGRATULATIONS TO YOU AND YOUR PARENTS. MAY GOD GRANT THEM THE JOY OF SEEING IN YOU THE REALIZATION OF ALL THEIR HOPES AND PRAYERS.

CONGRATULATIONS AND BEST WISHES ON THE DAY OF YOUR BAR MITZVAH.

Birthday:

A SIMPLE GREETING, SHORT AND SNAPPY, TO HOPE YOUR BIRTHDAY WILL BE HAPPY.

HAPPY BIRTHDAY. HERE'S WISHING YOU THE VERY BEST OF EVERYTHING, TODAY AND ALWAYS.

Births:

JUST ARRIVED . . . POUNDS . . . OUNCE(S) BOY (GIRL). MOTHER AND SON (DAUGHTER) DOING FINE. WANTED YOU TO BE ONE OF THE FIRST TO KNOW.

LOVE AND BEST WISHES TO BABY AND MOTHER. KNOW YOU ARE HAPPY TO WELCOME ANOTHER.

Bon Voyage:

BON VOYAGE. BEST WISHES FOR A PLEASANT TRIP AND A HAPPY LANDING.

BEST WISHES FOR A WONDERFUL TRIP AND A SAFE RETURN. WE'LL BE THINKING OF YOU ALL THE TIME.

Commencement:

CONGRATULATIONS. MAY YOUR DIPLOMA BE YOUR PASSPORT TO UNBOUNDED SUCCESS.

HEARTIEST CONGRATULATIONS. MAY ALL YOUR AMBITIONS BE REALIZED.

Communion:

MAY GOD'S BLESSINGS ON THIS HOLY COMMUNION DAY BE WITH YOU ALL THROUGH THE YEARS.

OUR HEARTS ARE FILLED WITH HAPPINESS FOR YOU ON YOUR FIRST HOLY COMMUNION DAY.

Condolences:

WE ARE GRIEVED BEYOND EXPRESSION TO LEARN OF YOUR GREAT LOSS. GOD BLESS AND COMFORT YOU.

WAS GREATLY SHOCKED AT THE SAD NEWS. YOU HAVE OUR (MY) DEEPEST SYMPATHY.

Confirmation:

OUR THOUGHTS AND PRAYERS ARE WITH YOU ON THIS YOUR CONFIRMATION DAY.

MAY GOD'S BLESSINGS ON THIS HOLY CONFIRMATION DAY BE MULTIPLIED THROUGHOUT THE YEARS.

Congratulations:

(on a promotion)

HEARTY CONGRATULATIONS ON YOUR PROMOTION. NO ONE EVER DESERVED IT MORE. GOOD LUCK AND THE BEST OF EVERYTHING.

HAPPY TO HEAR OF YOUR PROMOTION. HOPE IT IS JUST ONE OF MANY MORE TO COME. SINCERE CONGRATULATIONS.

(on election to office)

YOU FULLY DESERVE THE HONOR OF YOUR NEW OFFICE. CONGRATULATIONS AND THE BEST OF EVERYTHING.

OVERJOYED THAT YOU WON. PREDICT GREAT SUCCESS IN YOUR NEW OFFICE. CONGRATULATIONS.

(on having delivered a speech)

WELL DONE! YOUR EXCELLENT SPEECH WAS CONVINCING AND TO THE POINT.

CONGRATULATIONS ON A FINE SPEECH. I AM CONFIDENT IT HAS WON MANY NEW FRIENDS AND SUPPORTERS TO YOUR CAUSE.

(on opening a new business)

WITH ALL GOOD WISHES AND SUCCESS THAT EXCEEDS YOUR EXPECTATIONS. YOU DESERVE EVERY SUCCESS AND WE (I) KNOW YOU WILL HAVE IT.

(on winning a prize or award)

JUST A SMALL TRIBUTE TO THE WINNER OF THE . . . PRIZE (AWARD). HEARTIEST CONGRATULATIONS FOR THE WELL-EARNED RECOGNITION.

CONGRATULATIONS ON THE HIGH HONOR BESTOWED ON YOU. YOUR WORK DESERVES IT. EVERY CONTINUED SUCCESS.

(on the performance of a public service)

OUR RESPECT AND ADMIRATION GO OUT TO YOU AS A GREAT PUBLIC SERVANT. WE ALL APPLAUD YOUR STRAIGHTFORWARD ACTION.

IT'S MEN (WOMEN) LIKE YOU WHO ARE HELPING TO MAKE THIS COUNTRY A BETTER PLACE TO LIVE. CONGRATULATIONS.

(on an artistic success)

I WAS NEVER SO MOVED BY A PERFORMANCE. YOU WERE TRULY MAGNIFICENT. CONGRATULATIONS.

HEARTIEST CONGRATULATIONS ON YOUR HIGHLY SUCCESSFUL EXHIBIT (PHOTOGRAPHY, PAINTING, SCULPTURE, etc.).

Convalescence:

BEST WISHES FOR A SPEEDY RECOVERY AND ALL THE LUCK IN THE WORLD.

SORRY TO HEAR YOU HAVE BEEN ILL. MISS YOU AND HOPE YOU WILL BE BACK WITH US SOON. REGARDS FROM ALL.

Engagement:

DELIGHTED TO HEAR THE GOOD NEWS. CONGRATULATIONS AND EVERY HAPPINESS.

ENGAGEMENT IS WONDERFUL NEWS. LOVE AND HAPPINESS TO YOU BOTH AND BEST WISHES FOR A FUTURE FULL OF JOY.

Good Luck:

GOOD LUCK IN EVERYTHING YOU DO. YOU DESERVE THE BEST LIFE HAS TO OFFER.

GOOD LUCK TO YOU IN YOUR NEW HOME. MAY YOU ENJOY EVERY HAPPINESS FOR MANY YEARS.

Invitations:

HOPE YOU CAN MAKE OUR MEETING NEXT TUESDAY. EXPECT A BIG TURNOUT. PLANNING SOME WONDERFUL ENTERTAINMENT.

EXTENDING CORDIAL INVITATION TO HEAR TALK ON (subject) AT (place), ON (date and time). REFRESHMENTS.

New Years:

MAY THE NEW YEAR BRING YOU AND YOUR FAMILY A FULL MEASURE OF HEALTH, HAPPINESS AND PROSPERITY.

HAPPY NEW YEAR. MAY THE HAPPINESS CONTINUE FOR YOU AND YOURS ALL THROUGH THE YEAR.

Thanksgiving:

MAY YOUR HOME BE FULL OF HAPPINESS AND CHEER ON THANKSGIVING DAY AND EVERY DAY OF THE YEAR.

BEST WISHES FOR A HAPPY THANKSGIVING. YOU ARE MORE THAN EVER IN OUR THOUGHTS AT THIS TIME.

Thank you:

THANK YOU FOR YOUR LOVELY GIFT. IT WAS A DELIGHTFUL SURPRISE AND WILL BE SO USEFUL.

WE (I) CAN NEVER TELL YOU HOW TRULY GRATEFUL WE (I) ARE (AM) FOR YOUR HELP. NOTHING CAN TAKE THE PLACE OF A TRUE FRIEND. THANKS.

Wedding:

BLESSINGS ON YOUR WEDDING DAY. MAY YOUR ROAD THROUGH LIFE BE LIT WITH HAPPINESS AND JOY.

HEARTIEST CONGRATULATIONS. MAY ALL YOUR DAYS BE AS HAPPY AS THIS ONE.

INTERNATIONAL TELEGRAPH SERVICE

The international telex and telegram are the means by which written messages can be sent to overseas points or to ships at sea almost immediately.

There are two basic classes of international telegraph service that are of primary interest to the general public for commercial and social use. These are:

1. Full Rate Telegrams
2. Letter Telegrams

Full Rate Telegrams provide the fastest overseas service as they are accepted for immediate handling and transmission. The text may be written in plain language or code or both. There is a minimum charge for seven words.

Letter Telegrams, where accepted, provide a more economical overnight service. There is a minimum charge for 22 words at a rate half that for Full Rate Telegrams. If filed before midnight, they are generally delivered the next day. The text must be expressed wholly in plain language.

Format for international telegraph blanks

Blank telegraph forms are provided free by the major international communications carriers — RCA Global Communications, Inc.; ITT World Communications, Inc.; TRT

Telecommunications Corp.; and Western Union International, Inc. These forms provide space for indicating the following:

1. Type of service desired
2. Sender's name
3. Sender's address
4. Recipient's name
5. Street address (or registered code address)
6. City and country
7. Routing indicator (Via ITT, RCA, TRT or WUI)
8. Text or message
9. Signature (optional)

In filling out the telegraph form, it is preferable to type or print. Any international telegraph blank can be used to send overseas messages via any international carrier. The completed form may be filed at any Western Union public office or agency or at any office of the international telegraph carriers. Offices with Telex or TWX can readily send international Telex and telegrams via teletypewriter. International telegram messages may also be telephoned from home or office.

Preparing the telegraph form for transmission

The following are the essential steps in preparing the blank form for transmission:

1. Check the kind of service desired. Unless the sender indicates that it is a Letter Telegram, it is assumed that Full Rate service is desired.

2. Information in the preamble, such as word count, origin, date, filing time, etc., is generally completed by telegraph company personnel.

3. The name and address of the sender is placed in the appropriate space.

4. The recipient's name and address is placed in the space provided. The address must contain all necessary information to insure prompt delivery of the telegram. Registered code addresses, if available, should be used to reduce costs. There is no charge for the name of the country to which the message is being sent.

5. Your routing designation of one of the major international communications carriers should be placed after the address of destination. This will prevent delay caused by the domestic carrier having to process the international telegram through the "unrouted pool", and it will assure the greatest likelihood of one-carrier service at both ends of the transmission. There is no charge for such routing designation. (Via ITT designates ITT World Communications, Inc.; Via RCA designates RCA Global Communications, Inc.; Via WUI designates Western Union International, Inc.; Via TRT designates TRT Telecommunications Corp.)

6. The message should be clear and concise. Keep chargeable words to a minimum.

7. The signature is optional. If included, it is counted and charged for.

8. Although the sender's name and address are placed on the form, these are for reference purposes only and are not chargeable.

International Telegram Via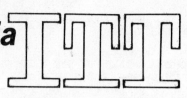

GEORGE BURKE
500 EAST 42 STREET
NEW YORK, N.Y. 10017
(2120 679 - 1595
Sender's Name and Address

Word Count_____ *Full Rate Unless Otherwise Checked (√)*

☒ *Full Rate*   ☐ *Letter Telegram Service (LT)*

Date   ☐ *Other (Specify)*

To   THOMAS REYNOLDS
     18 RUEDELAPAIX
     PARIS (FRANCE)

► ITT

insert "ITT"

If you send this blank to a Western Union
Telegraph office, insert ITT here. If you
telephone your message in, or use a desk fax
or teleprinter, insert Via ITT after the address.

BENSON ARRIVING TOMORROW STEAMER LIBERTE. PLS MEET ON ARRIVAL.

           BURKE

*All messages are accepted subject to rates, rules and regulations in the
applicable tariffs on file with the Federal Communications Commission.*

ITT World Communications Inc.

subsidiary of International Telephone and Telegraph Corporation

70

1. Is domestic service used only for the transmission of messages within the United States? Explain.

2. What are Mailgrams?

3. Which are the two basic types of delivery of telegrams?

4. Which class has no additional charge for physical delivery of the message?

5. List the essential steps in preparing a blank domestic telegraph form for transmission.

6. What other domestic telegraph services are available?

7. What are the two basic classes of international telegraph service?

8. Which class of international telegraph service provides the fastest service?

9. List the essential steps in preparing a blank international telegraph form for transmission.

10. What are the advantages of indicating the routing designation on an international telegram?

Good Grammar and Correct
Usage in Letter Writing

THE PARTS OF SPEECH

All the words in the English language are classified according to the way they are used in a particular sentence. These classifications are called the *parts of speech*. There are eight parts of speech: *nouns, pronouns, adjectives, verbs, adverbs, prepositions, conjunctions* and *interjections*.

Nouns

NOUNS are the names of persons, places, things or qualities.

The *student* sat in the *classroom*.

The *books* are here.

Courage is important.

CONCRETE NOUNS: Name persons, places or things which can be identified by sight, sound, smell, taste or touch.

automobile   noise   perfume   bread   crowd

ABSTRACT NOUNS: Name qualities or general ideas which cannot be identified by any of the five senses.

freedom   health   loyalty   wisdom

COMMON NOUNS: Name a kind or class of beings, places or things.

soldier   city   invention

PROPER NOUNS: Name some special or particular being, place, thing or event.

Thomas Edison   Broadway   New York Times   Easter

COLLECTIVE NOUNS: Name a group or collection of beings, places or things by using a singular form. Collective nouns may be either common or proper nouns.

Congress   jury   family   Senate

When such group or collection is considered as a unit, the collective noun is followed by a singular verb.

The whole family *was* invited.

When such group or collection is thought of as a number of individuals, the collective noun is followed by a plural verb.

The jury *were* unable to agree on a verdict.

Pronouns

PRONOUNS are used to take the place of nouns.

The guests arrived. *They* came early.

PERSONAL PRONOUNS show whether the person is speaking (first person); is spoken to (second person); or whether the person or thing is spoken about (third person).

The nominative forms of personal pronouns are used when the pronoun is the subject of the verb, or the complement of any form of the verb *to be*.

We visited the patient.

It is *I*.

Nominative forms:	Singular	Plural
1st Person:	I	we
2nd Person:	you	you
3rd Person:	he / she / it	they

The objective forms of personal pronouns are used when the pronoun is the object of a verb or of a preposition.

The girls saw *him*.

Give the magazine to *her*.

Objective forms:	Singular	Plural
1st Person:	me	us
2nd Person:	you	you
3rd Person:	him / her / it	**them**

REFLEXIVE and INTENSIVE PRONOUNS: Personal pronouns ending in *self* or *selves* have two uses — the *reflexive* use and the *intensive* use.

	Singular	Plural
1st Person:	myself	ourselves
2nd Person:	yourself	yourselves
3rd Person:	himself / herself / itself	themselves

When the pronoun is *reflexive*, it refers back to the subject. Unlike the intensive pronoun, it is separated from the subject for which it stands.

The player hurt *himself*.

When a pronoun is *intensive*, it emphasizes the noun or pronoun with which it is used. It generally follows immediately after the noun or pronoun which it intensifies.

He *himself* won the game.

RECIPROCAL PRONOUNS express a mutual relationship between or among individuals. The two reciprocal pronouns are *each other* and *one another*.

Arnold and Florence are very fond of *each other*.

POSSESSIVE PRONOUNS: Personal pronouns that show ownership or possession are called *possessive pronouns*:

The toys are *theirs*.
Are these tickets *ours*?

	Singular	*Plural*
1st Person:	mine	ours
2nd Person:	yours	yours
3rd Person:	his hers its	theirs

RELATIVE PRONOUNS relate or connect an adjective clause to the antecedent. The relative pronouns are **who, whom, whose, that** and **which**.

Use *who, whom* or *whose* when referring to persons only.

Who is the nominative form and is used when the pronoun is the subject of the verb or the complement of any form of the verb *to be*.

The man *who* telephoned is here.
I know *who* it is.

Whom is used when the pronoun is the object of and directly follows a preposition.

I know of *whom* you speak.

Either *who* or *whom* is acceptable when the pronoun is the object of a verb or a following preposition.

The man *who* you called is here.
The man *whom* you called is here.
I know *who* you gave it to.
I know *whom* you gave it to.

Whose is the possessive form and is used to show possession or ownership.

Betty is the girl *whose* parents you met.

That is generally used when referring to animals or things.

The horses *that* I saw belong to Jack.
The steaks *that* you bought are delicious.

That may also be used when referring to persons, as follows:

1. When referring to a word used in a superlative or exclusive sense.

She is the loveliest girl *that* I have met.

2. When referring back to both persons and things.

Where are the workmen and tools *that* we need?

Which is used only when referring to animals, places or things. However, *which* and *that* are frequently interchangeable.

The animal *which* he caught is a fox.
The land *which* he discovered was later named America.
The land *that* he discovered was later named America.
The letter *which* he expected was not received.
The letter *that* he expected was not received.

INTERROGATIVE PRONOUNS are used to introduce a question. The interrogative pronouns are *who, whom, whose, which* and *what*.

Use *who, whom* and *whose* when referring to persons.

Who is used when the pronoun is the subject of a verb or the complement of any form of the verb *to be*.

Who knocked at the door?
Who is it?

Either *who* or *whom* is acceptable when the pronoun is the object of a verb.

Who did you meet?
Whom did you meet?

Whom must be used when the pronoun is the object of a preposition.

To *whom* was it sent?

Whose is used as the possessive form.

Whose did you borrow?

Use *which* when selecting a particular being, place or thing.

You have a choice of pie or cake. *Which* do you want?

Use *what* when referring to things only.

What is the color of your new car?

DEMONSTRATIVE PRONOUNS point out persons, things or ideas. The singular forms are *this* and *that*. The plural forms are *these* and *those*.

I do not understand *that*.
These are the samples.

INDEFINITE PRONOUNS do not have a specific antecedent. They refer to certain individuals or things without specifying which ones.

The following indefinite pronouns are singular and take the singular verb form:

another	everybody	nothing
anybody	everyone	one
anyone	everything	somebody
anything	much	someone
each	neither	something
each one	no one	
either	nobody	

One of the men *was* hurt.
Neither of us *has* finished.

The following indefinite pronouns are plural and take the plural verb form:

both   few   many   others   several
Several are leaving now.

Each of the following indefinite pronouns may be either singular or plural, depending on its intended meaning in the sentence:

all   any   most   none   some

Most of the money *has* been spent.
Most of the students *know* him.

73

Adjectives

ADJECTIVES are used to modify nouns or pronouns.

> Gertrude is a *charming* girl.
> She is *tall*.

Adjectives are usually divided into two main classes — descriptive and limiting.

DESCRIPTIVE ADJECTIVES indicate the kind or condition of the words described. This is done by means of such qualities as color, size, shape, smell, taste, etc.

> *white* chalk   *large* house   *round* table   *sick* boy

LIMITING ADJECTIVES modify words without giving any information about the kind or condition of the words modified. Limiting adjectives may be subdivided into *possessive adjectives, demonstrative adjectives, numerical adjectives* and *article adjectives*.

Possessive adjectives show ownership or possession.
> *my* wife   *her* coat   *our* home   *his* friend

Demonstrative adjectives "point out" the nouns.
> *this* man   *these* men   *that* picture   *those* pictures

Numerical adjectives express a definite or indefinite amount or indicate the order in a series.
> *one* student   *double* portion
> *fifth* week   *several* years

Article adjectives consist of the definite and the indefinite articles.
> *the* tree   *a* bed   *an* apple

Verbs

Every sentence in the English language must contain a verb. Verbs are used to show action or a state of being.

> Mother *baked* the cake.
> Frank *hit* the ball.
> Ruth *is* ill.
> The child *slept* in the crib.

TRANSITIVE VERBS show an action that is received by someone or something.

> The hunter *shot* the deer.
> Kate *wrote* a long letter.

INTRANSITIVE VERBS express a state of being or action that is not received by anyone or anything.

> They *are* a happy couple.
> She *writes* well.

REGULAR VERBS form the past tense and past participle by adding *ed, d* or *t*. Most verbs in the English language are regular.

> *wash washed   love loved   deal dealt*

IRREGULAR VERBS form the past tense and past participle without adding *ed, d* or *t*. Most of the 200 irregular verbs form their past tense and past participle by a vowel change. A list of the principal parts of irregular verbs and other difficult verbs appears on pages 77-79.

Agreement of the verb with the subject

The verb must agree with the subject in both *person* and *number*. Failure to observe this rule is the cause of many errors in spoken and written English.

Person is the form or use of the verb which shows whether the subject is the speaker (first person); the person spoken to (second person); or the person or thing spoken about (third person).

Number is the form or use of the verb which shows whether the subject is one (singular) or more than one (plural).

1. Two or more subjects connected by *and* generally take a plural verb.

> Ralph and Betty *were* very angry.

However, a compound subject referring to a single person, or considered as a unit, takes a singular verb.

> My old friend and neighbor *is going* to Chicago.
> Bread and butter *was* Bobby's favorite food.

2. The word *there* may be used to introduce a sentence. However, it is not the subject but merely an introductory word. The verb following this introductory word should agree with the real subject which follows the verb.

> There *is* a man waiting at the door.
> There *are* many guests at the party.

3. Do not be confused by words that appear between the subject and the verb. The verb must always agree with the subject.

> A box of cigars *was* on the table.
> The stories in the magazine *are* interesting.

In the first sentence, the verb *was* agrees with the subject *box.* (singular) In the second sentence, the verb *are* agrees with the subject *stories.* (plural)

4. The addition of such expressions as *accompanied by, in addition to, as well as, together with*, etc., does not influence the number of the verb.

> Walter, as well as his friends, *enjoys* baseball.

In the example given above, the subject *Walter* is singular. The expression *as well as his friends* does not change the number of the subject. Hence, the singular form of the verb *enjoys* is correct.

5. If two singular subjects are joined by *either ... or* or *neither ... nor*, the verb is singular; if both subjects are plural the verb is plural.

> Either Miriam or Jean *is going* with you.
> Neither the boys nor the girls *were* late.

However, if one subject is singular and the other is plural, the verb must agree with the subject nearer the verb.

> Either my brothers or sister *is coming*.
> Neither my sister nor brothers *are coming*.

6. Collective nouns that are singular in meaning and in form take a singular verb. Some commonly used collective nouns are:

army	company	gang	nation
band	couple	group	navy
board	crowd	herd	orchestra
choir	department	jury	pair
class	enemy	majority	party
club	family	minority	squad
committee	firm	mob	team
community	flock		

The team *is* ready.
The crowd *was waiting*.

On occasion, the different members of a group are meant rather than the group as a whole. In such cases, the noun is plural in number and takes a plural verb.

The jury *were divided* in their thinking.

7. Use a singular verb with nouns that are plural in form but singular in meaning. Examples of such nouns are:

civics	mathematics	physics
economics	measles	politics
ethics	mumps	United States
gallows	news	whereabouts

The news *is* exciting.

A few such nouns are considered plural in meaning and take plural verbs. Examples of such words are:

pliers	scissors	trousers

His trousers *are torn*.

8. A subject that has to do with quantity, distance, time, number, etc., takes a singular verb when the subject is regarded as a unit.

Fifty dollars *is* a large sum of money.
Four plus four *is* eight.

If a fraction is followed by a singular object, the verb is singular; if it is followed by a plural object, the verb is plural.

One-half of the bottle *is* empty.
One-half of the bottles *are* empty.

The different moods of the verb

The *mood* of a verb indicates the manner in which the statement is made. The three different moods are *indicative*, *imperative* and *subjunctive*.

Indicative mood

The *indicative mood* is used to state a fact or ask a question. This mood is the one most often used in English.

Laura *dances* well.
How *are* the children?

Imperative mood

The *imperative mood* is used to make a request or to express a command. This mood is always in the second person (singular or plural) and in the present tense (the present infinitive form without *to*). The subject is *you* understood.

Halt!
Sit down.
Please shut the door.

Subjunctive mood

The *subjunctive mood* is not used frequently in current English. However, it is still used to express a wish, make a demand, or voice a condition contrary to fact.

The verb *to be* is the only one currently used in the subjunctive mood. Rarely, if ever, are any of the other verbs used in this way. *To be* has two common subjunctive forms: *be* is for all persons, singular or plural, in the present tense; *were* is used for all persons, singular or plural, in the past tense.

I demand that he *be* punished.
Raymond wished he *were* taller.
If I *were* you, I would buy the radio.

Use and formation of tenses

Present tense
(simple form)

This tense is used to express an ordinary action or condition.

I *eat* breakfast every morning.
The train *leaves* at noon.
She *is* a beautiful girl.
He *has* a new hat.

Except for the verb *to be*, most verbs in the present tense (simple form) are alike in the first and second person. The third person singular is usually formed by adding *s*. Some verbs, like *go, catch, box*, etc., form the third person by adding *es*. It should be noted that the third person singular of the verb *to have* is *has* (not *haves*).

Following is the conjugation of the verb *to be* in the simple form of the present tense:

	Singular	Plural
1st Person:	am	are
2nd Person:	are	are
3rd Person:	is	are

Present tense
(progressive form)

The progressive form of the present tense is used to express an action or condition that is going on in the present. It is obtained by using the present tense (simple form) of the verb *to be* with the present participle of the main verb.

She *is sleeping* now.
They *are sitting* in the park.
I *am writing* a letter.

Present tense
(emphatic form)

The emphatic form of the present tense *emphasizes* an ordinary action or condition. It is obtained by using the present tense (simple form) of the helping verb *to do*, followed by the present infinitive of the main verb.

You *do sing* well.
He *does understand* the lesson.

Present tense
(perfect form)

The present perfect tense expresses:
1. An action or condition that has just been completed
   She *has bought* a new dress.

2. An action or condition that began in the past and is still continuing in the present

He *has spoken* for ten minutes.

3. An indefinite or repeated action or condition that occurred in the past

I *have heard* that song before.
We *have been* there many times.

The present perfect tense is formed by using the present (simple form) of the verb *to have*, followed by the past participle of the main verb.

Past tense
(simple form)

The simple form of the past tense expresses an action or condition that was completed in the past:

We *had* a long vacation last year.
She *went* to the theatre yesterday.

Excluding the verb *to be*, all verb forms in the past tense (simple form) are alike for all persons.

Following is the conjugation of the verb *to be* in the past tense, simple form:

	Singular	*Plural*
1st Person:	was	were
2nd Person:	were	were
3rd Person:	was	were

Past tense
(progressive form)

The past tense progressive form shows an action or condition that was going on, or continuing, at a given moment in the past. It is obtained by using the past tense of the helping verb *to be*, followed by the present participle of the main verb.

I *was reading* when the bell rang.
When they arrived, we *were having* dessert.

Past tense
(emphatic form)

The past tense emphatic form emphasizes a past action or condition. It is obtained by using the past tense of the helping verb *to do*, followed by the present infinitive of the main verb.

I *did lend* you the money.
You *did have* a cold last week.

Past tense
(perfect form)

The past tense perfect form shows an action or condition that had occurred prior to some other past action or condition. It is formed by using the past tense of the helping verb *to have*, followed by the past participle of the main verb.

They came after the play *had begun*.

Future tense
(simple form)

The simple form of the future tense expresses an action or condition that is going to take place in the future. It is formed by using *will* as the helping verb followed by the present infinitive of the main verb.

We *will see* you tonight.
They *will be* home soon.
You *will meet* them next week.

Another way of expressing the simple form of the future tense is to use the progressive form of the present tense of the verb *to go*, followed by the infinitive of the main verb.

I *am going* to sell the house.
She *is going* to sweep the floor.

Future tense
(progressive form)

The progressive form of the future tense shows an action or condition that will be going on, or continuing, at a given moment in the future. It is obtained by using the future form of the helping verb *to be*, followed by the present participle of the main verb.

At noon tomorrow, the sun *will be shining*.
We *will be swimming* in the pool when you return.

Future tense
(perfect form)

The perfect form of the future tense expresses an action or condition that will be completed at some definite time in the future. It is formed by using the future tense of the helping verb *to have*, followed by the past participle of the main verb.

We *will have driven* 250 miles by midnight.
By 7 p.m., they *will have had* their dinner.

Principal parts of irregular and other special verbs

Present (Infinitive)	Past	Past Participle	Present Participle
(to) arise	arose	arisen	arising
be (am-are-is)	was-were	been	being
bear (produce)	bore	born	bearing
bear (carry)	bore	borne	bearing
beat	beat	beaten or beat	beating
become	became	become	becoming
begin	began	begun	beginning
behold	beheld	beheld	beholding
bend	bent	bent	bending
bid (order)	bade	bidden	bidding
bid (offer)	bid	bid	bidding
bind	bound	bound	binding
bite	bit	bitten	biting
bleed	bled	bled	bleeding
blow	blew	blown	blowing
break	broke	broken	breaking
breed	bred	bred	breeding
bring	brought	brought	bringing
build	built	built	building
burst	burst	burst	bursting
buy	bought	bought	buying
can	could	....	....
cast	cast	cast	casting
catch	caught	caught	catching
choose	chose	chosen	choosing
cling	clung	clung	clinging
come	came	come	coming
cost	cost	cost	costing
creep	crept	crept	creeping
cut	cut	cut	cutting
deal	dealt	dealt	dealing
dive	dived or dove	dived	diving
do	did	done	doing
draw	drew	drawn	drawing
drink	drank	drunk or drank	drinking
drive	drove	driven	driving
dwell	dwelt	dwelt	dwelling
eat	ate	eaten	eating
fall	fell	fallen	falling
feed	fed	fed	feeding
feel	felt	felt	feeling
fight	fought	fought	fighting
find	found	found	finding
flee	fled	fled	fleeing
fling	flung	flung	flinging
fly	flew	flown	flying
forbid	forbade or forbid	forbidden or forbid	forbidding
forget	forgot	forgotten or forgot	forgetting
forgive	forgave	forgiven	forgiving
forsake	forsook	forsaken	forsaking
freeze	froze	frozen	freezing
get	got	gotten or got	getting
give	gave	given	giving
go	went	gone	going

Present (Infinitive)	Past	Past Participle	Present Participle
(to) grind	ground	ground	grinding
grow	grew	grown	growing
hang	hung or hanged	hung or hanged	hanging
have	had	had	having
hear	heard	heard	hearing
hide	hid	hidden or hid	hiding
hit	hit	hit	hitting
hold	held	held	holding
hurt	hurt	hurt	hurting
keep	kept	kept	keeping
know	knew	known	knowing
lay (put)	laid	laid	laying
lead	led	led	leading
leave	left	left	leaving
lend	lent	lent	lending
let	let	let	letting
lie (rest)	lay	lain	lying
lose	lost	lost	losing
make	made	made	making
may	might	....	....
mean	meant	meant	meaning
meet	met	met	meeting
pay	paid	paid	paying
put	put	put	putting
read	read	read	reading
rend	rent	rent	rending
rid	rid or ridded	rid or ridded	ridding
ride	rode	ridden	riding
ring	rang	rung	ringing
rise	rose	risen	rising
run	ran	run	running
say	said	said	saying
see	saw	seen	seeing
seek	sought	sought	seeking
sell	sold	sold	selling
send	sent	sent	sending
set	set	set	setting
shake	shook	shaken	shaking
shed	shed	shed	shedding
shine (beam)	shone	shone	shining
shoot	shot	shot	shooting
shrink	shrank or shrunk	shrunk	shrinking
shut	shut	shut	shutting
sing	sang or sung	sung	singing
sink	sank or sunk	sunk	sinking
sit	sat	sat	sitting
slay	slew	slain	slaying
sleep	slept	slept	sleeping
slide	slid	slid	sliding
sling	slung	slung	slinging
slink	slunk	slunk	slinking
slit	slit	slit	slitting
speak	spoke	spoken	speaking
speed	sped or speeded	sped or speeded	speeding
spend	spent	spent	spending

Present (Infinitive)	Past	Past Participle	Present Participle
(to) spin	spun	spun	spinning
spit	spat or spit	spat or spit	spitting
split	split	split	splitting
spread	spread	spread	spreading
spring	sprang or sprung	sprung	springing
stand	stood	stood	standing
steal	stole	stolen	stealing
stick	stuck	stuck	sticking
sting	stung	stung	stinging
stride	strode	stridden	striding
strike	struck	struck or stricken	striking
string	strung	strung	stringing
strive	strove or strived	striven or strived	striving
swear	swore	sworn	swearing
sweep	swept	swept	sweeping
swim	swam	swum	swimming
swing	swung	swung	swinging
take	took	taken	taking
teach	taught	taught	teaching
tear	tore	torn	tearing
tell	told	told	telling
think	thought	thought	thinking
throw	threw	thrown	throwing
thrust	thrust	thrust	thrusting
understand	understood	understood	understanding
wear	wore	worn	wearing
weave	wove	woven	weaving
weep	wept	wept	weeping
win	won	won	winning
wind (twist)	wound	wound	winding
wring	wrung	wrung	wringing
write	wrote	written	writing

Adverbs

ADVERBS are used to modify verbs, adjectives or other adverbs.

> The girl ate *quickly*. (modifies verb *ate*)
> The room is *too* warm. (modifies adjective *warm*)
> He spoke *very* loudly. (modified adverb *loudly*)

There are adverbs of time, place, manner, degree and assent and dissent:

1. ADVERBS OF TIME answer the question: *When?*
   > They will arrive *tomorrow*.
   > Fred came *late*.

2. ADVERBS OF PLACE answer the question: *Where?*
   > The passengers went *ashore*.
   > She is standing *there*.

3. ADVERBS OF MANNER answer the question: *How?*
   > She speaks *well*.
   > Do it *slowly*.

4. ADVERBS OF DEGREE indicate extent and answer the question: *How much?*
   > You are *quite* correct.
   > Do it *more* carefully.

5. ADVERBS OF ASSENT present an affirmative answer and *adverbs of dissent* present a negative answer to a question.
   > *Yes*, you may have it.
   > *No*, I have not finished the book.

Prepositions

PREPOSITIONS are used to show the relationship between nouns or pronouns and other words in sentences.

> The boy walked *with* her *to* the park.

Some of the more commonly used prepositions are:

about	before	by	like	through
above	behind	down	near	to
across	below	during	of	toward
after	beneath	except	off	under
against	beside	for	on	underneath
along	besides	from	outside	until
among	between	in	over	up
around	beyond	inside	past	upon
at	but	into	since	with

Conjunctions

CONJUNCTIONS are used to connect words or groups of words.

> You *and* I must leave soon.
> I went to bed *because* I was tired.

Some of the more commonly used conjunctions are:

after	because	if	still	unless
also	but	nor	that	until
although	for	otherwise	therefore	when
and	hence	since	then	while
as	however	so	though	yet

Interjections

INTERJECTIONS are used to express sudden or intense feeling. They are merely exclamatory words and are not part of the main idea of a sentence. Interjections are used in conversation and in letters of a personal nature. They are seldom used in business correspondence.

> Ouch! It hurts.
> Well, return it tomorrow!

PHRASES, CLAUSES AND SENTENCES

We are now ready to study how the various parts of speech are used in phrases, clauses and sentences.

The phrase

A phrase is a group of words that presents an idea but does not express a complete thought and has no subject or predicate. A phrase may be used in a sentence as an adjective, an adverb or a noun. The four principal kinds of phrases are:

The PREPOSITIONAL PHRASE is a group of words introduced by a *preposition*. It can be used in a sentence as an adjective, adverb or noun.

> Your term *of office* is over. (adjective modifying the noun *term*)
> The letter will be sent *in a few days*. (adverb modifying the verb *sent*)
> The shot came *from across the street*. (noun, object of preposition *from*)

The PARTICIPIAL PHRASE is a group of words introduced by a participle. It can be used in a sentence only as an *adjective*.

> The promotion *given you* was well deserved (adjective modifying *promotion*)

The GERUND PHRASE is a group of words introduced by a gerund. (verbal noun). It can be used in a sentence only as a *noun*.

> *Swimming* daily is a healthful form of exercise. (noun, subject of verb *is*)

The INFINITIVE PHRASE is a group of words introduced by an *infinitive*. It can be used in a sentence as an adjective, adverb or noun.

> Did you make an attempt *to complete the report?* (adjective modifying the noun *attempt*)
> She left *to visit her sister*. (adverb modifying verb *left*)
> *To find the solution* requires careful effort. (noun, subject of verb *requires*)

The clause

A clause is a group of words which has both a subject and a predicate and which forms part of a sentence. The two kinds of clauses are: *main* or *independent clause* and *subordinate* or *dependent clause*.

The Main or Independent Clause is one that expresses a complete grammatical thought and may stand alone as a sentence. There may be one or more main clauses in a sentence.

We were elated when he received the promotion.
We will furnish the material, but *you must submit a requisition.*

The Subordinate or Dependent Clause contains a subject and a predicate but cannot stand alone. It depends upon the remainder of the sentence for its meaning. It can be used in the sentence as a noun, adjective or adverb.

The Noun Clause is a subordinate clause that is used in the sentence as a noun.

Whatever you say will be done. (subject of verb *will be done*)

The Adjective Clause is a subordinate clause that modifies a noun.

The salesman *whom you recently hired* is competent. (modifies noun *salesman*)

The Adverbial Clause is a subordinate clause that modifies a verb, adjective or other adverb.

We will pay the bill *when you deliver the merchandise.* (modifies the verb *pay*)
You are taller *than I am.* (modifies adjective *taller*)
Mr. Wilson speaks more distinctly *than you do.* (modifies the adverb *more distinctly*)

The sentence

A sentence is a group of words containing a subject and a predicate and expressing a complete thought. Sentences are classified according to meaning into three kinds: *declarative, interrogative* and *imperative.*

A Declarative Sentence is used to state something.

It is still raining.
He asked whether she had finished the report.

An Interrogative Sentence is used to ask a question.

Did you enjoy your vacation?

An Imperative Sentence is used to express a request or a command. *You,* understood, is the subject of an imperative sentence.

Please be quiet.
Halt!

Sentences expressing surprise or strong emotion are called *exclamatory sentences.* However, they must be either *declarative, interrogative* or *imperative.*

Wow! It hurts! (declarative)
Wasn't it terrible? (interrogative)
Watch out! (imperative)

Sentences are also classified according to structure into four kinds: *simple, compound, complex* and *compound-complex.*

A Simple Sentence is a sentence which contains only one main clause.

The package was delivered last night.

A Compound Sentence is a sentence which contains two or more main clauses.

Mother likes coffee but father prefers tea.

A Complex Sentence is a sentence which contains one main clause and one or more subordinate clauses.

We worked until the night shift arrived.
If she does well in her classwork and if she gets a high mark in the final test, Ruth may receive an "A" for the course.

A Compound-Complex Sentence is a sentence which contains two or more main clauses and one or more subordinate clauses.

They worked as quickly as possible to meet the deadline; but when the whistle blew, the work was still not finished.

Parts of the sentence

All sentences consist of two parts: the *subject* and the *predicate.*

The Subject is that part of the sentence about which something is said. In an interrogative sentence, the subject is that part about which something is asked.

The train stopped at the station.
Is *he* tall or short?
Do it now! (*you*)
Suddenly, *the lights* went out.

The Predicate is that part of the sentence that tells something about the subject.

The train *stopped at the station.*
Is he *tall or short?*
Do it now!

RULES OF SPELLING

There is one rule you should always follow: When in doubt about the spelling or the meaning of a word, consult a dictionary. There are several kinds of dictionaries: *abridged* and *unabridged.* The abridged dictionary contains fewer words and offers less information. The unabridged dictionary is not only larger but contains a great many more words and the information it offers is complete. Both kinds are authoritative and reliable. Whichever dictionary you use, keep it handy as your best "word friend."

Words with *ei* and *ie*

1. When the sound of the two vowels is a long *e*, place *i* before *e* except after *c*.

brief	field	niece	pier	relief
ceiling	conceit	conceive	deceive	receive

2. When the sound of the two vowels is not a long *e*, the *e* is usually placed before the *i*.

eight	heir	neighbor	rein

The exceptions to this rule are:

either	leisure	seize
financier	neither	weird

81

Final *e*

1. With most words ending in silent *e*, drop the *e* before a suffix that begins with a vowel.

argue	arrive	desire	guide	love
arguing	arrival	desirous	guidance	lovable

The exceptions to this rule are:

The *e* is retained after soft *c* and soft *g* (race, rage) when the suffix *-ous* or *-able* is added.

advantageous	manageable	peaceable
chargeable	marriageable	serviceable
courageous	noticeable	traceable
	outrageous	

The *e* is retained in the endings *ye*, *oe* or *ee* before adding the suffix *-ing*

agreeing	eyeing	seeing
canoeing	guaranteeing	shoeing
dyeing	hoeing	

2. With most words ending in silent *e*, do not drop the *e* before a suffix beginning with a consonant.

amusement	improvement	movement	sincerely
careful	likeness	purely	surely
hopeless	management	safety	useful

The exceptions to this rule are:

acknowledgment	duly	truly
argument	judgment	wholly
awful	ninth	wisdom

Final *y*

1. With most words ending in *y* preceded by a consonant, the final *y* is changed to *i* before every suffix except *ing*.

carry	carrier	carrying
copy	copied	copying
satisfy	satisfied	satisfying
study	studious	studying
try	tried	trying

The exceptions to this rule are:

baby	babyhood	
city	citylike	
dry	dryness	
lady	ladyship	
shy	shyly	shyness
sly	slyly	slyness
wry	wryly	wryness

2. With most words ending in *y* preceded by a vowel, the final *y* is not changed when adding a suffix.

annoy	joy	obey	sway
annoyance	joyous	obeyed	swaying

The exceptions to this rule are:

day	lay	pay	say	slay
daily	laid	paid	said	slain

Final Consonant (words of one syllable)

1. With most words of one syllable that end in a single consonant (except *x*) that is preceded by a single vowel, we double the final consonant before a suffix that begins with a vowel.

drop	fix	hot	slap	wit
dropped	fixed	hottest	slapping	witty

A word that is an exception to this rule is: *gas — gaseous*.

2. Do not double the final consonant before a suffix that begins with a consonant.

glad	man	hat	sin
gladness	manhood	hatless	sinful

Final Consonant (words of two or more syllables)

1. With words that are accented on the last syllable and that end in a single consonant (except *x*) that is preceded by a single vowel, we double the final consonant before a suffix that begins with a vowel.

admit	begin	occur	regret
admitted	beginning	occurrence	regrettable

2. With words that end in a single consonant that is preceded by a single vowel, but is *not* accented on the last syllable, we do *not* double the final consonant before a suffix that begins with a vowel.

cancel	credit	profit	travel
canceled	creditor	profitable	traveling

3. Do *not* double the final consonant before a suffix beginning with a consonant.

brother	profit	regret
brotherhood	profitless	regretful

4. Do *not* double the final consonant when it is preceded by two vowels.

air	appear	defeat	suit
aired	appeared	defeated	suitable

5. Do not double the final consonant with words ending in two consonants.

confirm	insert	stamp	perform
confirmed	inserting	stamping	performing

Words ending in *-cede*, *-ceed* and *-sede*

1. Only one word ends in *-sede*
   supersede

2. Only three words end in *-ceed*
   exceed   proceed   succeed

3. All other words in this group end in *-cede*
   accede   intercede   precede   recede   secede

Words ending in *-ise*, *-ize* and *-yze*

1. The following commonly used words end in *-ise*

advertise	compromise	enterprise	supervise
advise	despise	exercise	surmise
arise	devise	merchandise	surprise
comprise	disguise	revise	televise

2. The following commonly used words end in *-ize*.

apologize	criticize	notarize	summarize
authorize	economize	publicize	systematize
characterize	humanize	realize	

3. The following commonly used words end in *-yze*
   analyze   paralyze

OTHER TROUBLESOME WORDS

Certain words in the English language can be confusing. They are words that, while similar in spelling or pronunciation, have different meanings; or words that, while similar in meaning, are not spelled or pronounced in the same way.

Following are some of such troublesome words that you should study and know how to use correctly.

absorption (taking up)
adsorption (adhesion)

accede (yield)
exceed (surpass)

accent (stress)
ascent (rise)
assent (agree)

accept (receive)
except (omit)

access (admittance)
excess (too much)

ad (advertisement)
add (addition)

adapt (convert)
adopt (take as one's own)

addition (adding process)
edition (copies published at one time)

advice (noun)
advise (verb)

affect (influence or pretend)
effect (bring about or result)

aisle (passage)
isle (island)

all ready (prepared)
already (by this time)

allusion (reference)
illusion (deception)

altar (place of worship)
alter (change)

altogether (completely)
all together (as a group)

alumna (woman graduate)
alumnae (women graduates)
alumnus (graduate)
alumni (graduates)

among (with three or more)
between (with only two)

anecdote (amusing incident)
antidote (remedy for poison)

angel (spiritual being)
angle (geometric figure)

appraise (evaluate)
apprise (inform)

ascent (climbing)
assent (agreement)

a while (a short time)
awhile (for some time)

beat (surpass an opponent in a game)
win (gain a victory in a game)

berth (bed)
birth (being born)

beside (nearby)
besides (in addition to)

biannual (twice a year)
biennial (every two years)

boarder (one who boards)
border (edge)

born (birth)
borne (carried)

borrow (receive a loan)
lend, lent, lending (make a loan)
loan (that which one borrows or lends)

bouillon (soup)
bullion (metal)

breath (noun)
breathe (verb)

bring (action toward the speaker)
take (action away from the speaker)

calendar (time schedule)
calender (to make smooth and
  glossy)

can (ability, also permission)
may (permission)

canvas (cloth)
canvass (solicit)

capital (money, city)
capitol (building)
Capitol (meeting place of
  Congress)

carat (weight)
caret (omission mark)
carrot (vegetable)

choose (present)
chose (past)

cite (quote)
sight (vision)
site (location)

climactic (climax)
climatic (climate)

clothes (garments)
cloths (fabrics)

coarse (not fine)
course (path)

complement (complete)
compliment (praise)

confidentially (secretly)
confidently (with confidence)

conscience (moral goodness)
conscious (aware)

continual (repeated at
  intervals)
continuous (unceasing)

core (inside)
corps (group)
corpse (dead body)

correspondence (letters)
correspondents (writers)

costume (dress)
custom (manner)

council (assembly)
counsel (advise, advice)
consul (government official)

credible (believable)
creditable (praiseworthy)

dairy (milk establishment)
diary (personal record)

decent (proper)
descent (act of descending)
dissent (disagreement)

desert (dry area)
dessert (part of meal)

device (contrivance)
devise (invent)

die, died, dying (cease to live)
die, died, dieing (cut or stamp)
die (tool)
dye, dyed, dyeing (color)
dye (noun—color)

disburse (pay)
disperse (scatter)

discreet (prudent)
discrete (distinct)

dual (two)
duel (combat)

elicit (obtain)
illicit (illegal)

emersion (act of appearing)
immersion (act of dipping)

emigrant (one who goes from)
immigrant (one who comes into)

eminent (distinguished)
imminent (about to occur)

envelop (verb)
envelope (noun)

expose (verb)
exposé (noun)

faint (weak, cowardly)
feint (trick)

farther (distance)
further (additional)

fewer (smaller number)
less (smaller amount)

flair (aptitude)
flare (brilliant light)

formally (in a formal manner)
formerly (previously)

forth (forward)
fourth (4th)

good (adjective)
well (adverb)

gorilla (ape)
guerrilla (type of warfare)

84

healthful (capable of giving
health)
healthy (in a state of good
health)

hear (listen)
here (place)

holy (sacred)
wholly (entirely)

in (position inside)
into (movement from outside to
inside)

ingenious (skillful)
ingenuous (simple)

it's (contraction of *it is*)
its (possessive form for *it*)

interment (burial)
internment (detention)

know (have knowledge of)
no (negative)

lady (correlative of lord or
gentleman)
woman (adult female person)

later (opposite of earlier)
latter (opposite of former)

latest (most recent)
last (final)

lath (wood)
lathe (machine)

lead (metal)
led (guided)

learn (acquire knowledge)
teach (impart knowledge)

leave (get off, go away,
abandon)
let (allow or permit)

lie, lay, lain, lying (rest or
recline)
lay, laid, laying (place or put)

linage (lines)
lineage (ancestry)

liqueur (aromatic, alcoholic
liquor)
liquor (liquid substance)

loath (reluctant)
loathe (detest)

lose (verb—suffer a loss)
loose (adjective—not fastened)
loss (noun—that which is lost)

mantel (shelf)
mantle (cloak)

marital (marriage)
martial (military)

meteorology (weather)
metrology (weights and
measures)

miner (mine worker)
minor (not an adult)

new (recent)
novel (unusual)

ordinance (law)
ordnance (military)

over-all (including everything)
overall (outer garment)

passed (past tense of *pass*)
past (time gone by)

peace (freedom from war)
piece (portion)

peak (top)
peek (sly glance)

per cent ⎫ (used after numerals
percent ⎭ only)
percentage (not used after
numerals)

perquisite (privilege)
prerequisite (requirement)

personal (individual)
personnel (staff)

perspective (view)
prospective (expectant)

plain (simple, level area)
plane (tool, surface)

post card (mailing card requiring a stamp)
postal card (government mailing card with printed postage
stamp)

pour (allow to flow deliberately)
spill (allow to fall or flow
unintentionally)

practical (useful)
practicable (capable of being
used)

85

precedence (priority)
precedents (examples)

presence (opposite of absence)
presents (gifts)

principal (chief)
principle (basic doctrine)

profit (gain)
prophet (one who prophesies)

prophecy (noun)
prophesy (verb)

quiet (still)
quit (discontinue or surrender)
quite (wholly)

raise (elevate or lift)
rise (get up or move upward)

receipt (acknowledgment)
recipe (formula)

register (record)
registrar (keeper of record or
    register)

reign (rule)
rein (harness)

respectfully (with respect)
respectively (in order given)

rob (refers to person or place
    being deprived)
steal (refers to object being
    stolen)

role (part to be played)
roll (turn, that which is rolled
    up)

salvage (save)
selvage (edging)

set, setting (place)
sit, sat, sitting (rest)

sewage (waste)
sewerage (drain system)

shined (polished)
shone (glowed)
shown (displayed)

shudder (tremble)
shutter (screen)

some time (period of time)
sometime (point of time)
sometimes (at times)

spacious (space)
species (classification)
specious (plausible)

stand (in upright position)
stay (dwell or remain)

stationary (fixed)
stationery (writing material)

statue (sculpture)
stature (height)
statute (law)

therefor (for it)
therefore (consequently)

timber (wood)
timbre (tone)

to (preposition)
too (also)
two (2)

track (course, path)
tract (region)

troop (soldiers)
troupe (actors)

valance (drape)
valence (chemistry)

than (used in comparisons)
then (refers to time)

their (possessive form of *they*)
there (place)
they're (contraction of *they are*)

waive (relinquish a claim)
wave (move to and fro)

weak (not strong)
week (seven days)

weather (atmospheric
    conditions)
whether (if)

who's (contraction of *who is* or
    who has)
whose (possessive form of *who*)

you're (contraction of *you are*)
your (possessive form of *you*)

TRITE OR HACKNEYED WORDS AND EXPRESSIONS

Trite or hackneyed words and expressions are those that have lost their effectiveness through overuse. Avoid them. They indicate a lack of originality and can be a source of irritation to the reader and the listener. The use of such tired and overused words and expressions in both personal and business correspondence comes from the faulty habit of using too many words that are really not necessary to bring out your intended meaning.

Triteness in business correspondence can be avoided by writing clearly and directly. You can achieve such a style if you omit superfluous words from your letters and try to avoid trite or hackneyed expressions.

Trite Expression	Simplified
at the present time at this time at the present writing	now
at your earliest convenience at the earliest possible moment by return mail	immediately
in due course in the near future at an early date	soon
at all times	always
for a period of a (month)	for a (month)
until such time as	until
in the course of	during
it is requested that you we will appreciate it if	please
we extend our thanks thank you kindly	thanks
trusting that you will send	please send
your esteemed favor of	your letter of
your letter of recent date	your recent letter
attached find attached you will find attached hereto	attached is (are)
enclosed herewith enclosed please find enclosed you will find	enclosed is (are) or we enclose
our records show according to our records	we find
in compliance with your request	as requested
as a matter of fact	in fact
at the city of (Philadelphia)	at (Philadelphia)
the writer	I
costs the sum of	costs
in a satisfactory manner	satisfactorily
due to the fact that owing to the fact that	because

in view of the circumstances	as
in the event of	if
as a matter of fact	in fact
in regard to	about
we regret to advise	we are sorry

Certain business terms which were very popular many decades ago must not be used in modern correspondence. Acceptable substitutions can be made easily.

Instead of	Use
advise	inform, phone, tell
beg	(delete)
favor	letter, order
inst. or instant	name of present month
kindly	please
prox. or próximo	name of following month
same (referring to a thing)	it
ult. or ultimo	name of preceding month

RULES FOR DIVIDING WORDS

In writing, it is sometimes necessary to divide a word at the end of a line. Bear in mind the following rules for dividing words:

1. Use a hyphen to indicate that the word is divided.
   advan-tage   cheer-ful   lib-erty   sepa-rate

2. Place the hyphen at the end of the line. The hyphen is never placed at the beginning of the next line.

.... dictionary ....

3. Divide words only between syllables.
   fla-vor   impor-tant   mix-ture   prob-ably

4. Do not divide words of one syllable.
   friend   length   planned   walked

5. Do not divide words containing less than six letters.
   ago   idea   index   open

6. Do not separate a one-vowel syllable that appears at the beginning or at the end of a word.
   amount   already   bacteria   obedience

7. a. A one-vowel syllable within a word should not be carried over to the next line but should appear at the end of the first line, before the hyphen.
   compari-son   presi-dent   privi-lege   regu-lar

   b. However, if a word contains two one-vowel syllables that are adjacent to each other, the word may be divided between these two vowels.
   idi-omatic   gradu-ation   radi-ator

8. Two-letter prefixes such as *de, en, ex, il, im, in, ir, re, un, etc.,* may be separated from the rest of the word.
   il-legal   im-possible   in-convenient   re-unite

9. Other two-letter beginning syllables and two-letter final syllables should not be separated from the rest of the word.

democracy   political   sunken   territory

10. a. Double consonants can generally be divided.

drug-gist   mil-lion   pos-sible   thin-nest

b. However, when a suffix is added to a word that ends in a double consonant, divide the word before the suffix.

call-ing   full-est   pass-ing

11. a. Compound words should be divided only between their major parts.

businessman   schoolgirl   textbook
business-man   school-girl   text-book

b. If the words are already hyphenated, they should be divided only at the hyphen.

courts-martial   ex-president

12. Do not divide contractions.

doesn't   o'clock   shouldn't   they've

13. Do not divide amounts stated in figures.

$150,329 $2,476.85   361,292

14. Do not divide the proper name of a person or place.

Herman   Shirley   Dalton   Harvey
Denver   Maryland   Pittsburgh   Wisconsin

15. If possible, avoid dividing dates. If the date must be divided, separate the year from the day.

.... *October 12,*
1492 ....
Note that no hyphen is used in such separation.

16. If possible, avoid dividing street addresses. If the address must be divided, separate the name of the street from *Avenue, Street, etc.*

.... *2201 Victory*
Avenue ....
Again, note that no hyphen is used in such separation.

17. Do not divide the last word in a paragraph or on the page.

RULES OF PUNCTUATION

We use punctuation to separate words and phrases so as to make the meaning of sentences clearer. Punctuation marks and the rules for their use are more or less standardized. Learn them — they will help you to write better business letters.

The period (.)

1. The period is used to mark the end of a declarative or an imperative sentence:

He delivered the insured package.
Send a reply immediately.

2. The period is used to mark the end of an indirect question:

He asked whether the letter had been typed.

3. The period is used after a request made in the form of a question:

Will you please send us a signed copy by return mail.

4. The period is used after initials and after most abbreviations:

Chas. R.E. Jones Mr. Jr. A.D. U.N. C.O.D.

5. The period is used in decimals, to separate dollars from cents, and before cents when written alone:

3.1416 $2.98 $.69

6. Three periods (ellipsis) ... may be used to show an intentional omission from a sentence:

"Hold the paper firmly ... but be sure your hands are clean."

The question mark (?)

1. The question mark is used at the end of a direct question:

Did he deliver the mail?

2. The question mark, placed within parentheses, is used to express doubt or uncertainty:

She was born in 1918 (?).

3. The question mark is placed after each question in a series that is part of a single sentence:

What are the dimensions of a No. 10 envelope? Of a No. 6¾ envelope? Of a monarch envelope?

The exclamation point (!)

1. The exclamation point is used after a sentence that expresses great surprise or strong emotion. Such an exclamatory sentence may be declarative, interrogative or imperative:

It hurts!
Wasn't it terrible!
Watch out!

2. The exclamation point is used also after strong interjections:

Wow!
Congratulations!

3. The exclamation point may be used for emphasis:

Make your reservations now!

The comma (,)

The comma is used in more ways than any other of the punctuation marks. Some of the more common uses of the comma are:

1. The comma is used to separate the day of the week from the month, and the day of the month from the year:

Friday, June 14   September 23, 196....

2. The comma is used to separate the name of the city or town from the name of the state:

Chicago, Illinois   Scarsdale, New York

3. The comma is placed after the salutation in personal letters unless open punctuation is used:

Dear Ruth,   Dear Uncle George,

4. The comma is placed after the complimentary closing in both business and personal correspondence unless open punctuation is used:

5. The comma is used to separate words in a series:

Howard is tall, intelligent, handsome and wealthy.

6. The comma is used to separate two parts of a sentence

that are connected by a conjunction:

>I enjoy the seashore, but she likes the country.

7. The comma is used to separate the name of the person addressed from the rest of the sentence:

>Fred, hand me the newspaper.

8. The comma is used to identify one part of a sentence with another part:

>Mr. Smith, the teacher, will arrive shortly.

9. The comma is used to separate such introductory words as *Yes, No, Please, Thank you, Naturally,* etc., from the rest of the sentence:

>*Yes,* I delivered the package personally.

10. The comma is used after an introductory phrase or clause that is not in its natural order:

>For additional information about postal rates, consult your local post office.
>If you can make delivery on time, wire me immediately.

11. The comma is used to separate a weak interjection from the rest of the sentence:

>Well, let her retype the letter.

12. The comma is used to set off a direct quotation from the rest of the sentence:

>Nora said, "I'll see you tomorrow."
>"This building," said the guide, "is the tallest in the world."

13. The comma is generally used before *Inc.* and *Ltd.* in the name of a company or corporation:

>Larkin Dye Co., Inc.
>British Mills, Ltd.

14. The comma is used to separate two adjectives, each of which modifies the noun:

>Margaret is a brilliant, conscientious student.

15. The comma is used to set off transitional words in sentences:

>The matter, therefore, is still undecided.

16. The comma is used to separate the hundreds from the thousands, the thousands from the millions, etc., in numbers of more than four digits:

>1,786,905   54,128   1200

The semicolon (;)

1. The semicolon is used to separate two independent clauses when the conjunction is omitted:

>Open the door; the room is very warm.

2. The semicolon is used to separate two independent clauses joined by a conjunction but already containing the commas:

>After graduation, Peter visited England, France and Spain; but when the telegram reached him, he returned home immediately.

3. The semicolon is used to separate two clauses joined by adverbs such as *accordingly, also, for example, furthermore, however, otherwise, therefore,* etc.:

>I read the letter carefully; however, I could not understand the message.

4. The semicolon is used to separate a series of items that within themselves contain commas:

>We sent invitations to relatives in Akron, Ohio; Baltimore, Maryland; Dallas, Texas; Richmond, Virginia; San Francisco, California; and Seattle, Washington.

The colon (:)

1. The colon is placed after the salutation in business correspondence unless open punctuation is used.

>Dear Sir: Gentlemen:

2. The colon is used to introduce a number of items that are to follow:

>Business success requires the following: industry, intelligence, personality and vision.

3. The colon may be used to introduce a long quotation:

>In 1865, President Abraham Lincoln said: "With malice toward none, with charity for all, with firmness in the right, as God gives us to see the right, let us strive to finish the work we are in."

4. The colon is used to separate hours from minutes in expressing time:

>8:45 a.m.   5:30 p.m.

5. The colon is used to separate the initials of the person who dictated a letter from those of his secretary, in the identification line of business correspondence:

>SJW:bp

6. The colon is used in Biblical references to separate chapter from verse:

>Jeremiah 23:5

7. The colon is used to express *to* in proportions:

>3:1   6:5

8. The colon is used in bibliographies to separate the place of publication from the name of the publisher:

>Magill, Robert, *Modern Verse,* New York: Royal Press, Inc., 1967.

The dash (—)

1. The dash is used to indicate a sudden shift in thought:

>Shall we — can we — increase the club dues?

2. The dash is used to indicate an unfinished statement:

>The child asked, "Mother, may I go —"
>"You may not," interrupted the mother.

3. The dash may be used to obtain a pause before an important word or phrase at the end of a sentence:

>The secret of her success is — personality.

4. The dash may be used to separate a summary from a series of terms preceding it:

>The typewriter, paper, envelopes — these we shall need.

5. A long dash may be used to indicate the omission of letters in a name:

>Mr. B —— of New York is handling the case.

Quotation marks (" ")

1. Quotation marks are used to enclose a direct quotation:

>The engineer reported, "The highway is safe."
>"The ocean," she remarked, "is very turbulent."

2. When more than one paragraph is quoted, quotation marks are placed before each paragraph, and only at the close of the final paragraph:

> "The House of Representative shall be composed of members elected by the people for two years.
>
> "A Representative must be twenty-five years old, a citizen of the United States for seven years and must live in the state where he is elected."

3. Quotation marks are used to indicate titles of short stories, magazine articles, poems, etc.:

> His article, "Teaching Idioms and Idiomatic Expressions," appeared in *The Public School Adult Educator.*

Titles of books, newspapers and magazines are italicized when printed, and underlined when handwritten or typewritten. The use of full capitals without any underlining for typewritten or printed titles is also accepted practice.

4. Quotation marks are used to enclose words having special meaning:

> The foreman has excellent "know-how" of the work.

5. Single quotation marks are used to enclose a quotation within a quotation:

> The letter specified, "Please send your reply 'Special Delivery.' "

Parentheses ( )

1. Parentheses are used to enclose non-essential explanatory matter:

> In order to vote, citizens must meet age (21 years in most states) and residence requirements.

2. Parentheses are used to enclose figures that repeat written-out words:

> I am enclosing ten dollars ($10.00) with this letter.

3. Parentheses may be used to enclose figures or letters used to enumerate a series of items:

> The four essential human freedoms expressed in President Roosevelt's message were: (1) Freedom of speech, (2) Freedom of worship, (3) Freedom from want, and (4) Freedom from fear.

The hyphen (-)

1. The hyphen is used as a mark to divide a word at the end of a line:

> Revenue bills must originate in the House of Representatives.

2. The hyphen may be used to connect several words that serve as a single adjective preceding a noun:

> a yellow-green color
> a well-balanced diet

However, the hyphen is omitted when the first word of the modifier is an adverb that ends in *ly,* or when the qualifying words *follow* a noun:

> a freshly prepared solution
> the diet is well balanced

3. The hyphen is used with spelled-out compound numbers from twenty-one to ninety-nine, and with fractions:

> thirty-five   one hundred fifty-three
> one-fourth   two-thirds

4. The hyphen is used to avoid an awkward union between the prefix or suffix and the root of the word:

> re-enter   un-American
> semi-invalid   bell-like

5. The hyphen may be used with the prefixes all-, ex-, half-, quarter-, self-, and the suffix -elect.

> all-American   quarter-turn
> ex-soldier   self-reliance
> half-awake   President-elect

6. The hyphen is used with words or expressions of a compound nature:

> brother-in-law   know-it-all
> jack-of-all-trades middle-of-the-road

7. The hyphen is used when a capital letter is joined to a noun:

> B-flat   I-beam
> C-clamp   T-square
> F-sharp   U-turn
> H-bomb   X-ray

8. The hyphen may be used to indicate the extremes of a series of dates or numbers:

> The material may be found on pages 16-21.
> World War II, 1941-1945, was one of the costliest wars ever fought.

The apostrophe (')

1. The apostrophe is used to show the omission of a letter or letters in a contraction:

> we've   didn't   o'clock   Ass'n
> I'm   hasn't   '64   B'klyn

2. The apostrophe is added to plural nouns that end in *s* to show ownership or possession:

> babies'   sisters'   visitors'

3. The apostrophe *s* ('s) is added to all singular nouns and to plural nouns not ending in *s* to show ownership or possession:

> student's   boss's   children's
> boy's   princess's women's

4. The apostrophe *s* ('s) is used to indicate the plural of numerals, letters and symbols that are considered as words:

> 7's   Q's   1960's   C.O.D.'s
> 11's   T's   &'s   IOU's

5. The apostrophe *d* ('d) is used to form the past tense of coined words:

> O.K.'d   X'd out

Brackets [ ]

1. Brackets are used to enclose an incidental remark made by someone who is quoting someone else:

> "Nathan Hale said: 'I regret that I have but one life to lose [some claim it to be *give*] for my country.' "

The brace {

1. The brace is used to show the relationship of one line to a group of lines:

> 3rd person { he
>   { she
>   { it

Orville Wright ⎫
Wilbur Wright ⎬ inventors of the airplane

The dieresis (··)

1. The dieresis is used to show that the second of the two vowels is pronounced in the syllable following:

naïve   coördinate

The diagonal bar (/)

1. The diagonal bar is used in some standard abbreviations:

B/L (bill of lading)   c/o (care of)

2. The diagonal bar is placed between *and* and *or* to indicate that either may be used to convey the meaning:

and/or

3. The diagonal bar is used in fractions:

22/7   6-3/4   15-7/8

The ditto mark (")

1. The ditto mark is used in informal work to indicate that a word or letter above is to be repeated:

Trip to Chicago and return   1500 miles
"   " Seattle   "   "   4500   "

The cedilla (ç)

1. The cedilla is used to indicate that the letter *c* under which it is placed has a soft sound:

façade

The leader (............)

1. A leader is a series of dots used to help the eye follow the material from the beginning to the end of a line:

		Page
Citizenship	....	11
History	....	14
Government	....	33

The caret (^)

1. The caret is used to indicate the insertion of words, letters, figures, etc., that had previously been omitted:

the City of
The United Nations headquarters is in ^ New York.

RULES OF CAPITALIZATION

There are not many rules of capitalization and they are not difficult to learn. Following are the general rules for proper capitalization.

1. Capitalize the first word of every sentence:

My parents enjoyed the performance.
When are you leaving?
Stop!

2. Capitalize proper nouns and proper adjectives:

Ireland
Harvard
George Washington
They sailed on an English ship.
We had French wine with our dinner.
I like Italian olive oil on my salad.

However, do not capitalize words which were originally proper nouns or proper adjectives but have now become common nouns or common adjectives:

watt   ampere
manila paper   derby hat

3. Capitalize the names of persons, organizations, institutions, places, streets, avenues, buildings, parks, etc.:

Lewis Ward   Empire State Building
Maine   Eastman Kodak Company
Boston   Pine Street
American Red Cross   Central Park
Mississippi River

4. Capitalize the initials of a name:

R. T. Smith

5. Capitalize titles when used with proper names:

Aunt Rose   Mr. Collins
Queen Elizabeth   President Jones

6. Capitalize abbreviations of academic degrees:

A.B.   B.S.   M.D.   Ph.D.

7. Capitalize the first word of a direct quotation:

He said, "This letter must be mailed immediately."

8. Capitalize the days of the week, the months of the year and holidays:

Sunday   June   Thanksgiving Day   Easter

9. Capitalize the names of religious groups, political parties, races and languages:

Catholic   Democrat   Indian   Jewish
Protestant   Republican   Negro   Latin

10. Capitalize the names of the Deity or words that refer to the Bible:

God   the Almighty   Lord   New Testament

11. Capitalize the pronoun I and the interjection O:

It is I.
Help me, O Lord.

12. Capitalize the first and other important words in the title of a book or magazine. Conjunctions, prepositions or articles that are part of a title are not generally capitalized:

A Tale of Two Cities
Gift from the Sea
Engineering and Mining Journal

13. The use of full capital letters for titles of books and magazines is permissible:

A TALE OF TWO CITIES
GIFT FROM THE SEA
ENGINEERING AND MINING JOURNAL

14. Capitalize the first words of lines of poetry:

By the rude bridge that arched the flood,
Their flag to April's breeze unfurled,
Here once the embattled farmers stood
And fired the shot heard 'round the world.

15. Do not capitalize the names of the seasons:

summer   fall   winter   spring

16. Do not capitalize words indicating direction unless they refer to geographic regions:

Drive *north* for two miles and turn *east*.
They will visit the Far East and the South Pacific.

THE USE OF CONTRACTIONS

Although contractions are not recommended for formal styles of writing, they are used in general conversation and in informal correspondence such as personal letters.

Use the apostrophe (') in contractions at the exact place where the letters, words or figures are omitted. Periods are not required, as contractions are not abbreviations.

association	here is	let us	of the clock	secretary	1973
ass'n	here's	let's	o'clock	sec'y	'73

Pronouns with "am," "are" and "is":

I am	I'm	we are	we're
you are	you're	you are	you're
he is	he's	they are	they're
she is	she's	these are	these're
it is	it's	those are	those're
that is	that's		
what is	what's		
who is	who's		

Pronouns with "have" and "has":

I have	I've	we have	we've
you have	you've	you have	you've
he has	he's	they have	they've
she has	she's	these have	these've
it has	it's	those have	those've
who has	who's	who have	who've
that has	that's		

Pronouns with "shall" and "will":

I'll	she'll	this'll	we'll
you'll	it'll	who'll	you'll
he'll	that'll	which'll	they'll
			these'll
			those'll

Pronouns with "had," "should" and "would":

I'd you'd he'd she'd who'd we'd you'd they'd

Negatives: (*Ain't* should *not* be used for *am not*)

are not	aren't	is not	isn't
can not	can't	must not	mustn't
could not	couldn't	need not	needn't
did not	didn't	shall not	shan't
do not	don't	should not	shouldn't
does not	doesn't	was not	wasn't
had not	hadn't	we're not	weren't
has not	hasn't	will not	won't
have not	haven't	would not	wouldn't

Miscellaneous Information

SPECIAL FORMS OF ADDRESS FOR OFFICIALS

Good usage requires that the proper form of address be used in correspondence with government officials, members of the armed forces, members of the clergy and many others whose title or position requires a special identifying form of address.

The degree of formality in such correspondence varies. It depends on the relationship between the writer and the official, as well as the subject matter of the letter. Where, in addressing an official, you do not know the full name or are not certain of the spelling of the name, it is proper to address the letter to the official position, or the office the person holds. A letter addressed in this way requires a more formal salutation and complimentary closing than that addressed to a particular person. On the whole, a less formal style is favored in most official correspondence.

Following is a comprehensive listing of the many different forms of official address. Refer to it whenever you have occasion to correspond with someone who holds an official post.

| Envelope and Inside Address | Salutation | Complimentary Closing |

PUBLIC OFFICIALS

(Federal)

The President of the United States

| The President
The White House
Washington, D. C. 20500 | Sir:
My dear Mr. President:
Dear Mr. President: | Respectfully,
Respectfully yours,
Respectfully yours, |

Wife of the President

| Mrs. (name in full)
The White House
Washington, D. C. 20500 | Dear Mrs. ....: | Sincerely yours, |

The Vice-President of the United States

| The Honorable (name in full)
The Vice-President of the United States
Washington, D. C. 20501 | Sir:
Dear Sir:
Dear Mr. Vice-President:
Dear Mr. ....: | Very truly yours,
Very truly yours,
Sincerely yours,
Sincerely yours, |

The President of the Senate

| The Honorable (name in full)
President of the Senate
Washington, D. C. 20510 | Dear Sir:
My dear Mr. President:
Dear Mr. President: | Very truly yours,
Very truly yours,
Sincerely yours, |

The District of Columbia abbreviation (D.C.) used in addresses in this section has been in general use for many years in business letter writing. The special two-letter abbreviation authorized by the U.S. Postal Service for use with the ZIP Code for the District of Columbia is DC.

President pro tempore of the Senate

The Honorable (name in full)   Dear Sir: Very truly yours,
President pro tempore of the Senate   Dear Senator: Sincerely yours,
United States Senate   Dear Senator ....:   Sincerely yours,
Washington, D. C. 20510

Senator

The Honorable (name in full)   Dear Sir (Madam):   Very truly yours,
The United States Senate   My dear Senator ....:   Sincerely yours,
Washington, D. C. 20510   Dear Senator ....:   Sincerely yours,

Speaker of the House of Representatives

The Honorable (name in full)   Dear Sir (Madam):   Very truly yours,
Speaker of the House of Representatives   Dear Mr. (Madam) Speaker: Sincerely yours,
Washington, D. C. 20515   Dear Mr. (Madam) ....:   Sincerely yours,

Member of Congress

The Honorable (name in full)   Dear Sir (Madam):   Very truly yours,
The House of Representatives   My dear Congressman
Washington, D. C. 20515   (Congresswoman) ....:   Sincerely yours,
                                      My dear Mr. (Madam) ....:   Sincerely yours,
                                      Dear Mr. (Madam) ....:   Sincerely yours,

Cabinet Member

The Honorable (name in full)   Dear Sir (Madam):   Very truly yours,
Secretary of (department)   My dear Mr. (Madam)
Washington, D. C.   (ZIP Code number)   Secretary ....:   Very truly yours,
                                      Dear Secretary: Sincerely yours,
                                      Dear Mr. (Madam) ....:   Sincerely yours,

Chief Justice of the United States

The Honorable (name in full)   My dear Mr. Chief Justice: Very truly yours,
Chief Justice of the United States   Dear Mr. Chief Justice: Very truly yours,
Washington, D. C. 20543

Associate Justice of the United States Supreme Court

The Honorable (name in full)
Justice of the Supreme Court of the   My dear Mr. Justice: Very truly yours,
   United States   Dear Mr. (Madam) Justice: Sincerely yours,
Washington, D. C. 20543

(International)

American Ambassador

The Honorable (name in full)   Sir (Madam):   Very truly yours,
American Ambassador   Dear Mr. (Madam)   Sincerely yours,
City, Country   Ambassador:

Secretary General of the United Nations

His Excellency (name in full)
Secretary General of the United Nations
New York, New York   10016

Excellency:
Dear Mr. Secretary General:
Dear Mr. ....:

Very truly yours,
Sincerely yours,
Sincerely yours,

United States Representative to the United Nations

The Honorable (name in full)
United States Representative to
   the United Nations
New York, New York   10016

Sir:
Dear Mr. ....:

Very truly yours,
Sincerely yours,

Former President

The Honorable (name in full)
(local address) (ZIP Code Number)

Dear Mr. President:

Respectfully yours,

(State)

Governor of the State

The Honorable (name in full)
Governor of (name of state)
(state capital), State (ZIP Code number)

Sir (Madam):
Dear Sir (Madam):
My dear Governor ....:

Respectfully,
Respectfully yours,
Very truly yours,

Lieutenant Governor of State

The Honorable (name in full)
Lieutenant Governor of (name of state)
(state capital), State (ZIP Code number)

Sir (Madam):
Dear Sir (Madam):
Dear Mr. (Madam) ....:

Respectfully yours,
Very truly yours,
Sincerely yours,

State Senator

The Honorable (name in full)
State Senator
(state capital), State   (ZIP Code number)

Dear Sir (Madam):
Dear Senator ....:

Very truly yours,
Sincerely yours,

State Assemblyperson

The Honorable (name in full)
State Assemblyman (Assemblywoman)
(state capital), State   (ZIP Code number)

Dear Sir (Madam):
Dear Mr. (Madam) ....:

Very truly yours,
Sincerely yours,

Secretary of State

The Honorable (name in full)
Secretary of State of (name of state)
(state capital), State   (ZIP Code number)

Dear Sir (Madam):
My dear Mr. (Madam) ....:
Dear Mr. (Madam) ....:

Very truly yours,
Sincerely yours,
Sincerely yours,

Former Governor

The Honorable (name in full)
(local address)   (ZIP Code Number)

Dear Governor ....:

Sincerely yours,

(Municipal)

Mayor

The Honorable (name in full)　　　　Dear Sir (Madam):　　　　Very truly yours,
Mayor of (name of city)　　　　Dear Mr. (Madam) Mayor:　　　　Very truly yours,
(name of city), State　(ZIP Code number)

City Councilperson

Councilman (Councilwoman) (name in full)　　Dear Sir (Madam):　　　Very truly yours,
City Hall　　　　Dear Mr. (Madam) ....:　　　Sincerely yours,
(name of city), State　(ZIP Code number)

Commissioner of a City Department

The Honorable (name in full)　　　Dear Sir (Madam):　　　Very truly yours,
Commissioner of (name of department)　　Dear Commissioner ....:　　Sincerely yours,
(street address)　　　　Dear Mr. (Madam) ....:　　Sincerely yours,
(name of city), State　(ZIP Code number)

Former Mayor

The Honorable (name in full)
(local address)　(ZIP Code number)　　　Dear Mayor ....:　　Sincerely yours,

SCHOOL OFFICIALS AND FACULTY

President (with doctoral degree)

(name in full), (initials of degree)　　　Dear Sir (Madam):　　　Very truly yours,
President, (name of institution)　　　Dear Dr. ....:　　Sincerely yours,
(followed by postal address)

President (without doctoral degree)

Mr. (Madam) (name in full)　　　Dear Sir (Madam):　　　Very truly yours,
President, (name of institution)　　Dear Mr. (Madam) ....:　　Sincerely yours,
(followed by postal address)

Dean (with doctoral degree)

(name in full), (initials of degree)　　Dear Dean ....:　　Sincerely yours,
Dean, (name of school)　　　　Dear Dr. ....:　　Sincerely yours,
(name of institution)
(followed by postal address)

Dean (without doctoral degree)

Mr. (Madam) (name in full)　　　Dear Dean ....:　　Sincerely yours,
Dean, (name of school)　　　Dear Mr. (Madam) ....:　　Sincerely yours,
(name of institution)
(followed by postal address)

Professor (with doctoral degree)

(name in full), (initials of degree)   Dear Professor ....:   Sincerely yours,
(name of department)   Dear Dr. ....:   Sincerely yours,
(name of institution)
(followed by postal address)

Professor (without doctoral degree)

Professor (name in full)   Dear Professor ....:   Sincerely yours,
(name of department)
(name of institution)
(followed by postal address)

Associate Professor or Assistant Professor (with doctoral degree)

(name in full), (initials of degree)   Dear Professor ....:   Sincerely yours,
Associate (Assistant) Professor   Dear Dr. ....:
(name of department)
(name of institution)
(followed by postal address)

Associate Professor or Assistant Professor (without doctoral degree)

Mr. (Madam) (name in full)   Dear Professor ....:   Sincerely yours,
Associate (Assistant) Professor
(name of department)
(name of institution)
(followed by postal address)

Instructor

Dr. (name in full)   Dear Dr. ....:   Sincerely yours,
        or   Dear Mr. (Madam) ....:   Sincerely yours,
Mr. (Madam) (name in full)
(name of department)
(name of university)
(followed by postal address)

Superintendent of Schools

Dr. (name in full)   My dear Dr. ....:   Sincerely yours,
        or   My dear Mr. (Madam) ....:   Sincerely yours,
Mr. (Madam) (name in full)
Superintendent of Schools
(name of school system)
(followed by postal address)

School Principal

Dr. (name in full)   My dear Dr. ....:   Sincerely yours,
        or   My dear Mr. (Madam) ....:   Sincerely yours,
Mr. (Madam) (name in full)
Principal of (name of school)
(followed by postal address)

School Teacher

Envelope and Inside Address	Salutation	Complimentary Closing
Dr. (name in full) or Mr. (Madam) (name in full) (name of school) (followed by postal address)	Dear Dr. ....: Dear Mr. (Madam) ....:	Sincerely yours, Sincerely yours,

MEMBERS OF THE CLERGY

(Catholic)

Envelope and Inside Address	Salutation	Complimentary Closing
The Pope His Holiness, the Pope or His Holiness, Pope (name) Vatican City Italy	Your Holiness: Most Holy Father:	Respectfully yours,
Cardinal His Eminence (given name), Cardinal (surname) Archbishop of (diocese) (followed by postal address)	Your Eminence: My dear Cardinal ....:	Respectfully yours, Sincerely yours,
Archbishop The Most Reverend (name in full) Archbishop of (locality) (followed by postal address)	Your Excellency: My dear Archbishop: Dear Archbishop ....:	Respectfully yours, Respectfully, Sincerely yours,
Bishop The Most Reverend (name in full) Bishop of (locality) (followed by postal address)	Your Excellency: My dear Bishop: My dear Bishop ....:	Respectfully yours, Respectfully, Respectfully, Sincerely yours,
Monsignor (higher rank) The Right Reverend Monsignor (name in full) (followed by postal address)	Right Reverend Monsignor: My dear Monsignor: My dear Monsignor ....:	Respectfully yours, Respectfully, Sincerely yours,
Monsignor The Very Reverend Monsignor (name in full) (followed by postal address)	Very Reverend Monsignor: Dear Monsignor ....:	Respectfully, Sincerely yours,
Priest The Reverend (name in full) (followed by postal address)	Dear Father: Dear Father ....: Dear Dr. ....:	Respectfully, Sincerely yours, Sincerely yours,

Mother Superior
The Reverend Mother (name in full)
(followed by postal address)

Reverend Mother:
My dear Mother Superior:
Dear Mother ....:

Respectfully yours,
Respectfully,
Sincerely yours,

Sister
Sister (name in full)
(followed by postal address)

My dear Sister:
Dear Sister ....:

Respectfully yours,
Sincerely yours,

(Protestant)

Protestant Episcopal Bishop
The Right Reverend (name in full)
Bishop of (locality)
(followed by postal address)

Right Reverend Sir:
My dear Bishop:
My dear Bishop ....:

Respectfully yours,
Respectfully,
Sincerely yours,

Protestant Episcopal Dean
The Very Reverend (name in full)
Dean of (locality)
(followed by postal address)

Very Reverend Sir:
My dear Dean:
My dear Dean ....:

Respectfully yours,
Very truly yours,
Sincerely yours,

Methodist Bishop
The Reverend (name in full)
Methodist Bishop of (locality)
(followed by postal address)

Reverend Sir:
Dear Bishop ....:

Respectfully yours,
Sincerely yours,

Protestant Minister
The Reverend (name in full)
    or
Reverend (name in full), D.D.
Title, (name of church)
(followed by postal address)

Dear Sir:
My dear Mr. ....:
My dear Dr. ....:

Respectfully yours,
Sincerely yours,
Sincerely yours,

Mormon Bishop
Mr. (name in full)
Church of Jesus Christ of
    Latter Day Saints
(followed by postal address)

Sir:
Dear Mr. ....:

Respectfully,
Sincerely yours,

(Jewish)

Rabbi (name in full)
    or
Dr. (name in full)
(followed by postal address)

Dear Sir (Madam):
My dear Rabbi ....:
My dear Dr. ....:

Respectfully yours,
Sincerely yours,
Sincerely yours,

(Chaplain)

Chaplain (grade) (name in full)
(P.O. address of organization
    and station)

Dear Chaplain ....:

Sincerely yours,

MEMBERS OF THE ARMED FORCES

Correspondence to members of the armed forces must contain the complete address, including the exact title or rank, full name, and complete military or naval address (branch of service, unit, station or ship, etc.). In the salutation, the surname is placed in the blank space.

Rank or Rating and Abbreviation	Salutation	Complimentary Closing
(Army)		
O-10 General (GEN) O-9 Lieutenant General (LTG) O-8 Major General (MG) O-7 Brigadier General (BG)	Sir (Madam): Dear General: My dear General ....: Dear General ....:	Very truly yours, Very truly yours, Sincerely yours, Sincerely yours,
O-6 Colonel (COL) O-5 Lieutenant Colonel (LTC)	Dear Sir (Madam): Dear Colonel: My dear Colonel ....: Dear Colonel ....:	Very truly yours, Very truly yours, Sincerely yours, Sincerely yours,
O-4 Major (MAJ)	Dear Sir (Madam): Dear Major: My dear Major ....: Dear Major ....:	Very truly yours, Very truly yours, Sincerely yours, Sincerely yours,
O-3 Captain (CPT)	Dear Captain: My dear Captain ....: Dear Captain ....:	Very truly yours, Sincerely yours, Sincerely yours,
O-2 First Lieutenant (1LT) O-1 Second Lieutenant (2LT)	Dear Lieutenant: My dear Lieutenant ....: Dear Lieutenant ....:	Very truly yours, Sincerely yours, Sincerely yours,
W-4 Chief Warrant Officer (CW4) W-3 Chief Warrant Officer (CW3) W-2 Chief Warrant Officer (CW2) W-1 Warrant Officer (WO1)	Dear Mr. ....: Dear Mrs. ....: Dear Miss ....: Dear Ms. ....:	Sincerely yours, Sincerely yours, Sincerely yours, Sincerely yours,
E-9 Command Sergeant Major (CSM) E-9 Staff Sergeant Major (SSM) E-9 Sergeant Major (SGM)	Dear Sergeant Major: Dear Sergeant Major ....:	Very truly yours, Sincerely yours,
E-8 First Sergeant (1SG)	Dear First Sergeant: Dear First Sergeant ....:	Very truly yours, Sincerely yours,
E-8 Master Sergeant (MSG)	Dear Master Sergeant: Dear Master Sergeant ....:	Very truly yours, Sincerely yours,
E-7 Platoon Sergeant (PSG)	Dear Platoon Sergeant: Dear Platoon Sergeant ....:	Very truly yours, Sincerely yours,
E-7 Sergeant First Class (SFC)	Dear Sergeant First Class: Dear Sergeant First Class ....:	Very truly yours, Sincerely yours,
E-7 Specialist Seven (SP7)	Dear Specialist: Dear Specialist ....:	Very truly yours, Sincerely yours,
E-6 Staff Sergeant (SSG)	Dear Staff Sergeant: Dear Staff Sergeant ....:	Very truly yours, Sincerely yours,

Rank or Rating and Abbreviation		Salutation	Complimentary Closing
E-6	Specialist Six (SP6)	Dear Specialist: Dear Specialist ....:	Very truly yours, Sincerely yours,
E-5	Sergeant (SGT)	Dear Sergeant: Dear Sergeant ....:	Very truly yours, Sincerely yours,
E-5	Specialist Five (SP5)	Dear Specialist: Dear Specialist ....:	Very truly yours, Sincerely yours,
E-4	Corporal CPL)	Dear Corporal: Dear Corporal ....:	Very truly yours, Sincerely yours,
E-4	Specialist Four (SP4)	Dear Specialist: Dear Specialist ....:	Very truly yours, Sincerely yours,
E-3 E-2 E-1	Private First Class (PFC) Private (PV2) Private (PV1)	Dear Private: Dear Private ....:	Very truly yours, Sincerely yours,

(Air Force)

O-10 O-9 O-8 O-7	General (GEN) Lieutenant General (LtGen) Major General (MajGen) Brigadier General (BGen)	Sir (Madam): Dear General: My dear General ....: Dear General ....:	Very truly yours, Very truly yours, Sincerely yours, Sincerely yours,
O-6 O-5	Colonel (Col) Lieutenant Colonel (LtCol)	Dear Sir (Madam): Dear Colonel: My dear Colonel ....: Dear Colonel ....:	Very truly yours, Very truly yours, Sincerely yours, Sincerely yours,
O-4	Major (Maj)	Dear Sir (Madam): Dear Major: My dear Major ....: Dear Major ....:	Very truly yours, Very truly yours, Sincerely yours, Sincerely yours,
O-3	Captain (Capt)	Dear Captain: My dear Captain ....: Dear Captain ....:	Very truly yours, Sincerely yours, Sincerely yours,
O-2 O-1	First Lieutenant (1stLt) Second Lieutenant (2ndLt)	Dear Lieutenant: My dear Lieutenant ....: Dear Lieutenant ....:	Very truly yours, Sincerely yours, Sincerely yours,
W-4 W-3 W-2 W-1	Chief Warrant Officer (CWO-4) Chief Warrant Officer (CWO-3) Chief Warrant Officer (CWO-2) Warrant Officer (WO)	Dear Mr. ....: Dear Mrs. ....: Dear Miss ....: Dear Ms. ....:	Sincerely yours, Sincerely yours, Sincerely yours, Sincerely yours,
E-9	Chief Master Sergeant (CMSgt)	Dear Chief Master Sergeant: Dear Chief Master Sergeant ....:	Very truly yours, Sincerely yours,
E-8	Senior Master Sergeant (SMSgt)	Dear Senior Master Sergeant: Dear Senior Master Sergeant ....:	Very truly yours, Sincerely yours,

Rank or Rating and Abbreviation		Salutation	Complimentary Closing
E-7	Master Sergeant (MSgt)	Dear Master Sergeant: Dear Master Sergeant ....:	Very truly yours, Sincerely yours,
E-6	Technical Sergeant (TSgt)	Dear Technical Sergeant: Dear Technical Sergeant ....:	Very truly yours, Sincerely yours,
E-5	Staff Sergeant (SSgt)	Dear Staff Sergeant: Dear Staff Sergeant ....:	Very truly yours, Sincerely yours,
E-4	Sergeant (Sgt)	Dear Sergeant: Dear Sergeant ....:	Very truly yours, Sincerely yours,
E-4	Senior Airman (SrA)	Dear Senior Airman: Dear Senior Airman ....:	Very truly yours, Sincerely yours,
E-3 E-2 E-1	Airman First Class (A1C) Airman (Amn) Airman Basic (AB)	Dear Airman: Dear Airman ....:	Very truly yours, Sincerely yours,

(Marine Corps)

O-10 O-9 O-8 O-7	General (Gen) Lieutenant General (LtGen) Major General (MajGen) Brigadier General (BrigGen)	Sir (Madam): Dear General: My dear General ....: Dear General ....:	Very truly yours, Very truly yours, Sincerely yours, Sincerely yours,
O-6 O-5	Colonel (Col) Lieutenant Colonel (LtCol)	Dear Sir (Madam): Dear Colonel: My dear Colonel ....: Dear Colonel ....:	Very truly yours, Very truly yours, Sincerely yours, Sincerely yours,
O-4	Major (Maj)	Dear Sir (Madam): Dear Major: My dear Major ....: Dear Major ....:	Very truly yours, Very truly yours, Sincerely yours, Sincerely yours,
O-3	Captain (Capt)	Dear Captain: My dear Captain ....: Dear Captain ....:	Very truly yours, Sincerely yours, Sincerely yours,
O-2 O-1	First Lieutenant (1stLt) Second Lieutenant (2dLt)	Dear Lieutenant: My dear Lieutenant ....: Dear Lieutenant ....:	Very truly yours, Sincerely yours, Sincerely yours,
W-4 W-3 W-2 W-1	Chief Warrant Officer (CWO4) Chief Warrant Officer (CWO3) Chief Warrant Officer (CWO2) Warrant Officer (WO)	Dear Mr. ....: Dears Mrs. ....: Dear Miss ....: Dear Ms. ....:	Sincerely yours, Sincerely yours, Sincerely yours, Sincerely yours,
E-9	Sergeant Major (SgtMaj)	Dear Sergeant Major: Dear Sergeant Major ....:	Very truly yours, Sincerely yours,

		Salutation	Complimentary Closing
E-9	Master Gunnery Sergeant (MGySgt)	Dear Master Gunnery Sergeant:	Very truly yours,
		Dear Master Gunnery Sergeant ....:	Sincerely yours,
E-8	First Sergeant (1stSgt)	Dear First Sergeant:	Very truly yours,
		Dear First Sergeant ....:	Sincerely yours,
E-8	Master Sergeant (MSgt)	Dear Master Sergeant:	Very truly yours,
		Dear Master Sergeant ....:	Sincerely yours,
E-7	Gunnery Sergeant (GySgt)	Dear Gunnery Sergeant:	Very truly yours,
		Dear Gunnery Sergeant ....:	Sincerely yours,
E-6	Staff Sergeant (SSgt)	Dear Staff Sergeant:	Very truly yours,
		Dear Staff Sergeant ....:	Sincerely yours,
E-5	Sergeant (Sgt)	Dear Sergeant:	Very truly yours,
		Dear Sergeant ....:	Sincerely yours,
E-4	Corporal (Cpl)	Dear Corporal:	Very truly yours,
E-3	Lance Corporal (LCpl)	Dear Corporal ....:	Sincerely yours,
E-2	Private First Class (PFC)	Dear Private:	Very truly yours,
E-1	Private (Pvt)	Dear Private ....:	Sincerely yours,

(Navy and Coast Guard)

		Salutation	Complimentary Closing
O-10	Admiral (ADM)	Sir (Madam):	Very truly yours,
O-9	Vice Admiral (VADM)	Dear Admiral:	Very truly yours,
O-8	Rear Admiral (RADM)	My dear Admiral ....:	Sincerely yours,
		Dear Admiral ....:	Sincerely yours,
O-6	Captain (CAPT)	Dear Sir (Madam):	Very truly yours,
		Dear Captain:	Very truly yours,
		My dear Captain ....:	Sincerely yours,
		Dear Captain ....:	Sincerely yours,
O-5	Commander (CDR)	Dear Sir (Madam):	Very truly yours,
		Dear Commander:	Very truly yours,
		My dear Commander ....:	Sincerely yours,
		Dear Commander ....:	Sincerely yours,
O-4	Lieutenant Commander (LCDR)	Dear Sir (Madam):	Very truly yours,
		Dear Commander:	Very truly yours,
		My dear Commander ....:	Sincerely yours,
		Dear Commander ....:	Sincerely yours,

Rank or Rating and Abbreviation		Salutation	Complimentary Closing
O-3	Lieutenant (LT)	Dear Lieutenant:	Very truly yours,
O-2	Lieutenant Junior Grade (LTJG)	My dear Lieutenant ....:	Sincerely yours,
		Dear Lieutenant ....:	Sincerely yours,
O-1	Ensign (ENS)	Dear Ensign:	Very truly yours,
		My dear Ensign ....:	Sincerely yours,
		Dear Ensign ....:	Sincerely yours,
W-4	Chief Warrant Officer (CWO-4)	Dear Mr. ....:	Sincerely yours,
W-3	Chief Warrant Officer (CWO-3)	Dear Mrs. ....:	Sincerely yours,
W-2	Chief Warrant Officer (CWO-2)	Dear Miss ....:	Sincerely yours,
W-1	Warrant Officer (WO-1)	Dear Ms. ....:	Sincerely yours,
E-9	Master Chief Petty Officer (MCPO)	Dear Master Chief Petty Officer:	Very truly yours,
		Dear Master Chief Petty Officer ....:	Sincerely yours,
E-8	Senior Chief Petty Officer (SCPO)	Dear Senior Chief Petty Officer:	Very truly yours,
		Dear Senior Chief Petty Officer ....:	Sincerely yours,
E-7	Chief Petty Officer (CPO)	Dear Chief Petty Officer:	Very truly yours,
		Dear Chief Petty Officer ....:	Sincerely yours,
E-6	Petty Officer First Class (PO1)	Dear Petty Officer:	Very truly yours,
E-5	Petty Officer Second Class (PO2)	Dear Petty Officer ....:	
E-4	Petty Officer Third Class (PO3)		Sincerely yours,
E-3	Seaman (SN)	Dear Seaman:	Very truly yours,
E-2	Seaman Apprentice (SA)	Dear Seaman ....:	Sincerely yours,
E-1	Seaman Recruit (SR)		

ABBREVIATIONS OF THE STATES, THE DISTRICT OF COLUMBIA AND POSSESSIONS OF THE UNITED STATES

The following special 2-letter abbreviations have been authorized by the U.S. Postal Service for use with the ZIP Code. Use these special 2-letter abbreviations or the previously approved abbreviations noted in parentheses after the names of the states, possessions and the District of Columbia.

	Special 2-letter Abbreviations for Use with ZIP Code		*Special 2-letter Abbreviations for Use with ZIP Code*
Alabama (Ala.)	AL	New Jersey (N.J.)	NJ
Alaska	AK	New Mexico (N. Mex.)	NM
Arizona (Ariz.)	AZ	New York (N.Y.)	NY
Arkansas (Ark.)	AR	North Carolina (N.C.)	NC
California (Calif.)	CA	North Dakota (N. Dak.)	ND
Colorado (Colo.)	CO	Ohio	OH
Connecticut (Conn.)	CT	Oklahoma (Okla.)	OK
Delaware (Del.)	DE	Oregon (Oreg.)	OR
Florida (Fla.)	FL	Pennsylvania (Pa.)	PA
Georgia (Ga.)	GA	Rhode Island (R.I.)	RI
Hawaii	HI	South Carolina (S.C.)	SC
Idaho	ID	South Dakota (S. Dak.)	SD
Illinois (Ill.)	IL	Tennessee (Tenn.)	TN
Indiana (Ind.)	IN	Texas (Tex.)	TX
Iowa	IA	Utah	UT
Kansas (Kans.)	KS	Vermont (Vt.)	VT
Kentucky (Ky.)	KY	Virginia (Va.)	VA
Louisiana (La.)	LA	Washington (Wash.)	WA
Maine	ME	West Virginia (W. Va.)	WV
Maryland (Md.)	MD	Wisconsin (Wis.)	WI
Massachusetts (Mass.)	MA	Wyoming (Wyo.)	WY
Michigan (Mich.)	MI		
Minnesota (Minn.)	MN	Canal Zone (C.Z.)	CZ
Mississippi (Miss.)	MS	Guam	GU
Missouri (Mo.)	MO	Puerto Rico (P.R.)	PR
Montana (Mont.)	MT	Virgin Islands (V.I.)	VI
Nebraska (Nebr.)	NB		
Nevada (Nev.)	NV	District of Columbia	
New Hampshire (N.H.)	NH	(D.C.)	DC

abbr., abbrev.	abbreviation, abbreviated		c/o	care of
a.c.	alternating current		C.O.D.	cash on delivery
actg.	acting		coml.	commercial
A.D.	in the year of our Lord		comm.	commission, committee
ad, advt.	advertisement		Corp.	Corporation
ADP	Automatic Data Processing		C.P.A.	Certified Public Accountant
AFL-CIO	American Federation of Labor and Congress of Industrial Organizations		CPI	Consumer Price Index
			cr.	credit, creditor
			C.S.T.	Central Standard Time
Aly	Alley		Ct.	Court
a.m.	before noon		ctn.	carton
Am.	American		Ctr.	Center
amt.	amount		cu.	cubic
anon.	anonymous		cu.ft.	cubic foot
approx.	approximately		cu.yd.	cubic yard
Apr.	April		cwt	hundredweight
apt.	apartment			
Arc.	Arcade		d.c.	direct current
assn.	association		D.D.	Doctor of Divinity
assoc.	associate		D.D.S.	Doctor of Dental Surgery
asst.	assistant		Dec.	December
attn.	attention		deg.	degree, degrees
Atty.	Attorney		del.	deliver, delivery
Aug.	August		Dem.	Democrat
avdp.	avoirdupois		dept.	department
Ave., Av.	Avenue		dia., diam.	diameter
			diag.	diagonal, diagram
bal.	balance		dm	decimeter
bbl.	barrel		dol	dollar
B.C.	before Christ		doz	dozen
B/E	bill of exchange		dr.	debit, debtor
B/L	bill of lading		Dr.	Doctor, Drive
bldg.	building		D.S.T.	Daylight Saving Time
Blvd.	Boulevard		dtd.	dated
Bro(s).	Brother(s)		dz.	dozen
B/S	bill of sale			
bu	bushel		E.	East
bul.	bulletin		ea.	each
bx.	box, boxes		ed.	edition, editor
			e.g.	for example
C	centigrade, Celsius		enc., encl.	enclosure
cc, c.c.	carbon copy		Eng.	English
cc	cubic centimeter		env.	envelope
cf.	compare		e.o.m.	end of month
ch., chap.	chapter		Esq.	Esquire
Cir.	Circle		E.S.T.	Eastern Standard Time
cm	centimeter		et al.	and others
cm²	square centimeter		et seq.	and the following
cm³	cubic centimeter		etc.	and so forth
cml.	commercial		exch.	exchange
Co.	Company		exec.	executive

exp.	expense, export, express	K	karat
Expy.	Expressway	kc	kilocycle, kilocycles
Ext.	Extended, Extension	kg	kilogram
		km	kilometer
F	Fahrenheit	km²	square kilometer
F.A.S.	free alongside ship	km³	cubic kilometer
F.B.I.	Federal Bureau of Investigation	kt.	carat, kiloton
fbm	board foot	kw.	kilowatt
Feb.	February		
Fed.	Federal		
fig.	figure	l	liter
fl. oz.	fluid ounce, fluid ounces	La.	Lane
F.O.B.	free on board	lat.	latitude
Fri.	Friday	lb	pound
frt.	freight	L/C	letter of credit
Ft.	Fort	l.c.l.	less than a carload lot
ft	feet, foot	LL.D.	Doctor of Laws
Frwy.	Freeway	long.	longitude
fwd	forward	L.S.	place of the seal
F.Y.I.	for your information	Ltd.	Limited
g	gram, grams		
gal.	gallon, gallons	m.	meter, noon
Gdns.	Gardens	M	thousand
gi.	gill, gills	max.	maximum
Gov.	Governor	M.D.	Doctor of Medicine
govt.	government	mdse.	merchandise
gr.wt.	gross weight	memo	memorandum
		Messrs.	plural for Mr.
Hon.	Honorable	mfg.	manufacturing
hosp.	hospital	mfr.	manufacturer
h.p., hp	horsepower	mg	milligram
hr.	hour	Mgr.	Manager, Monsignor
Hts.	Heights	mi	mile, miles
Hwy.	Highway	min	minute, minutes
		misc.	miscellaneous
ibid.	in the same place	ml	milliliter
id.	the same	Mlle.	Mademoiselle
i.e.	that is	mm	millimeter
in	inch, inches	mm²	square millimeter
Inc.	Incorporated	mm³	cubic millimeter
init.	initial	Mme.	Madame
Inst.	Institute	mo.	month
inv.	invoice	Mon.	Monday
IOU	I owe you	m.p.h.	miles per hour
IQ	intelligence quotient	Mr.	Mister
ital.	italic, italics	Mrs.	Mistress, Madam
		Ms.	Miss or Mrs.
Jan.	January	msg	message
Jct.	Junction	M.S.T.	Mountain Standard Time
J.D.	Doctor of Laws (Juris Doctor)	Mt.	Mount, Mountain
jour.	journal	mtge.	mortgage
Jr.	Junior	mun.	municipal

N.	North
Natl.	National
N.B.	note carefully
N.D., n.d.	no date
n/f	no funds
No.	number
Nov.	November
nt.wt.	net weight
obit.	obituary
Oct.	October
O.K.	all correct, approved
o.s.	out of stock
oz	ounce
p., pp.	page, pages
par.	paragraph
pd.	paid
Ph.D.	Doctor of Philosophy
Pk.	Park
pkg.	package
Pkway.	Parkway
Pl.	Place
Plz.	Plaza
p.m.	afternoon
P.O.	post office
ppd.	prepaid
p.p.m.	parts per million
pr.	pair
Pres.	President
pro tem	temporarily
Prof.	Professor
P.S.	postscript
P.S.T.	Pacific Standard Time
pt.	part, point
pt	pint
q.	question
qt.	quart
quot.	quotation
Rd.	Road
recd.	received
Rep.	Republican
Rev.	Reverend
R.F.D.	Rural Free Delivery
rm.	ream, room
rms.	reams, rooms
R.N.	registered nurse
r/min.	revolutions per minute
r.p.m.	revolutions per minute

R.R.	Railroad, Right Reverend
R.S.V.P.	please reply
Ry.	Railway
S.	South
Sat.	Saturday
sec.	second
secy.	secretary
Sept.	September
shpt.	shipment
SOS	radio distress signal
Sq.	Square
Sr.	Senior
S.S.	Steamship
St.	Saint, Street
std.	standard
subj.	subject
Sun.	Sunday
Supt.	Superintendent
tbsp.	tablespoon
tech.	technical
tel.	telegram, telephone
temp.	temperature, temporary
Ter.	Terrace
terr.	territory
Thurs.	Thursday
Trl.	Trail
Treas.	Treasurer
tsp	teaspoonful
Tues.	Tuesday
Tpke.	Turnpike
TV	television
twp.	township
TWX	teletypewriter exchange
U.N.	United Nations
U.S.A.	United States of America
Via.	Viaduct
vid.	see
VIP	very important person
viz.	namely
vol.	volume
vols.	volumes
vou.	voucher
V.P.	Vice-President
vs.	versus, verse
v.v.	vice versa
W.	West
WATS	wide area telephone service
Wed.	Wednesday

wk.	week		yd²	square yard
wkly.	weekly		yd³	cubic yard
wt.	weight		yr	year
yd	yard		ZIP	Zone Improvement Plan

COMMONLY USED SIGNS AND SYMBOLS

+	plus		&	and
−	minus		@	at
±	plus or minus		*	asterisk
×	multiplied by		%	percent
·	multiplied by		$	dollars
÷	divided by		¢	cents
=	equal to		°	degree
≠	not equal to		′	minute, foot, feet
≡	identical with		″	second, inch, inches, ditto
>	greater than		#	number, pounds
≧	greater than or equal to		→	yields, direction of flow
<	less than		∡	angle
≦	less than or equal to		π	pi
:	is to, ratio		℞	take
::	as, proportion		©	copyright
∴	therefore		®	registered trademark
∵	because		√	square root
∝	varies as		a/c	account of
∞	infinity		á	acute accent
0	zero		à	grave accent
//	parallel		●	new moon
⊥	perpendicular		☽	first quarter
∟	right angle		○	full moon
△	triangle		☾	last quarter
□	square		♂	male
▭	rectangle		♀	female
▱	parallelogram		☠	poison
○	circle		✔	check
⌒	arc of circle		∧	caret